PSYCHOLOGY IN THE DENTAL OFFICE

TABLE OF CONTENTS

RESPONSIVE LISTENING

TALKING WITH PATIENTS

SPECIAL PATIENTS AND SITUATIONS

SECTION THREE: WORKING WELL TOGETHER -- THE DENTAL HEALTH TEAM

PSYCHOLOGY IN THE DENTAL OFFICE

INSTRUCTIONAL OBJECTIVES

THE STUDENT WILL BE ABLE TO:

1. Identify the oldest emotionally active part of the body.

2. List two of the three ways in which the teeth increase a child's capabilities and power.

3. List three of the four less commonly recognized ways in which the mouth and teeth are important to the adult.

4. List two of the three ways in which loss of teeth is threatening to the patient.

5. Identify three of the five motivational factors which affect patient behavior.

6. Describe how the need for acceptance and respect are affected by illness or a stress situation.

7. Compare the level of social adjustment described by the terms psychotic, neurotic and normal.

8. Describe three behavior traits of the "normal" dental patient.

9. List three of the five variables which affect the psychological perception of pain.

10. Describe how mild dental fears can affect treatment.

11. Describe two ways in which extreme dental fears may affect the patient's well-being.

12. Describe the body's flight-or-fight response to physical or emotional stress.

13. List three of the five defense mechanisms discussed.

14. Describe two of the three changes in the patient's behavior which occur when he trusts those treating him.

15. Describe two of the three things discussed that do not happen when you are concentrating on listening to the patient.

16. Identify one type each of those responses that do not help, that are neutral, and that do help.

17. Identify at least three roadblocks to communication.

18. State two of the three things you must do to send your message clearly.

19. Supply a better word which can be substituted for the following: pain, pull, fill, operatory, waiting room.

20. State three of the six given points to remember in giving instructions to a patient.

21. State one way in which we can give the patient a greater sense of controlling the dental situation and one way in which deployment may be used.

22. Describe the purpose of having a child make his first visit to the dentist before he has a toothache.

23. Describe two things which the exodontia patient may confuse with pain.

24. Describe two things which the auxiliary can do to help the elderly patient.

25. List two of the three major factors which are important in team building.

26. Identify the following by matching terms and definitions.*

affiliation	flight-or-fight response	psychology
anxiety	irrelevant statement	psychotic
control	mutilation	reflective listening
cultural bias	neurotic	regression
defense mechanisms	normal	repression
deployment	pain	socioeconomic
empathy	pain perception	stress
evaluative statement	pain threshold	supportive response
fear	philosophy of individual worth	you-message

* these terms are all included in the glossary at the end of this unit.

SECTION ONE: UNDERSTANDING THE DENTAL PATIENT

In this section we talk about some of the psychological factors which affect the dental patient's behavior. The discussion centers on accepting
the patient as a whole person and not regarding him merely as a set of teeth
to be fixed.

The emphasis is on the distressed patient and the factors which disturb him.
The topics covered in this section include: basic psychological implications
of the mouth and teeth; understanding and accepting patient behavior; psychotic,
neurotic and normal behavior; pain; fear and anxiety; and stress.

This information is necessary for our understanding of the problems which face
these patients; however, we should also remember that the majority of patients
encountered in the average dental practice are normal in their responses, cooperative during treatment, and pleasant people to be with.

SECTION TWO: HELPING THE DENTAL PATIENT

In this section we discuss ways in which we can use our understanding of the
patient to help him overcome his fears and anxieties about dentistry. We
deal in concrete ways in which you, the dental auxiliary, can work in cooperation with the dentist to help the patient be more comfortable and have a
better dental experience.

The major topics covered are: trust building; responsive listening; talking with patients; and special patients and situations.

SECTION THREE: WORKING WELL TOGETHER -- THE DENTAL HEALTH TEAM

The first two sections were devoted to understanding and helping the dental
patient. This one deals with the problems facing the dental health team
members in their relationships with each other.

The topics included are: stress and the dental health team; what can we
do to reduce this stress?; team building; and problem solving skills.

SECTION ONE: UNDERSTANDING THE DENTAL PATIENT

WHY LEARN ABOUT PSYCHOLOGY?

PSYCHOLOGY can be defined as, "The
science of the mind or mental states."

DENTISTRY is, "The health science
and art concerned with the care
and health of all tissues comprising the mouth."

There doesn't seem to be much con-
nection between these two sciences
until you remember that the tissues
comprising the mouth are surrounded
by, and an important part of, a
whole person complete with all of
the comlexities of human nature.

When a patient comes to the dental
office he brings with him all of
the feelings and emotions, previous
experiences and prejudices, strengths
and weaknesses which make him a
unique individual.

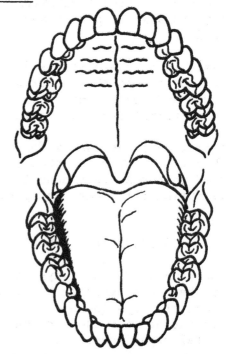

*PEOPLE BRING HUMAN FEELINGS TO THE
DENTAL CHAIR AS WELL AS THEIR TEETH!*

M. Massler

If we are to serve the whole patient, and not only the teeth, then we must
know something about people. According to Cinotti and Grieder[1], we can benefit from the study of psychology in two ways.

First: We may be helped to better understand our own feelings, motivations
and behavior. This can lead to improved effectiveness in dealing
with our own problems and in our relationships with others.

Second: Understanding the patient's feelings, motivation and behavior
enables us to be more accepting of him as a person and to provide better dental care.

INFANCY AND CHILDHOOD

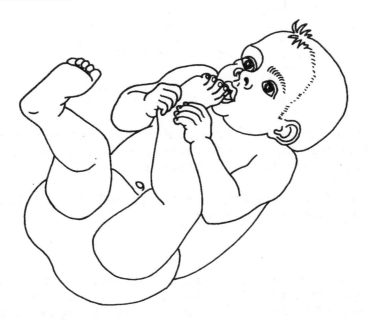

The mouth represents the oldest emotionally active part of the body as well as one of the most sensitive parts.

From the very beginning of life the mouth serves as the portal of communication between the individual and his world.

The newborn instinctively nuzzles and sucks to obtain the food he needs for survival. His first efforts at communication are his cries of hunger or discomfort. Later, as he begins to explore his world, he puts fingers, toys and toes into his mouth. He also learns that sucking his thumb or pacifier is a source of great comfort.

When teething starts, the child often has pain in the very area from which he has previously derived so much pleasure.[2] However, the eruption of the teeth involves an enormous increase in capabilities and power.

> The teeth are a new aid in obtaining nourishment.
> Now the child can bite and chew many foods.
>
> The child's communication skills increase
> markedly as he learns to talk.
>
> The child can express anger and hostility
> by biting and spitting. Thus he has increased
> ability to control and to harm.

ADULTHOOD

We use the mouth to communicate; to express aggression; as a sensual organ; as a very important stress-relieving mechanism, and, of course, for chewing.

People view the mouth as a very sacred part of the body -- and yet, this is where the dentist must intrude.

Alex Koper[3]

The mouth continues to be important throughout the life of the individual. This is demonstrated by the functions of eating, speaking, singing, love-making, etc. which it fulfills through adulthood.

The following are some of the less commonly recognized ways in which the mouth and teeth are important to the adult.

1. Power and Aggression

    The early use of the mouth as an instrument of aggression takes the form of biting and spitting. In the adult, however, aggressive speech constitutes one of the most socially acceptable forms of expressing anger and hostility.

    Also, many expressions and customs make it apparent that if we really wish to threaten a person physically we are prone to attack his mouth. An example of this is the bully who says,

    "I'LL KNOCK YOUR TEETH RIGHT DOWN YOUR THROAT!"

2. Self-Image

    Badly decayed, discolored or malpositioned teeth can severely affect the individual's self-image and psychological adjustment.

    *   Have you ever known someone with large protruding anterior teeth who was teased and called "Bugs Bunny"?

    *   Have you ever known someone with such badly decayed teeth that he never smiled for fear of having those teeth show? Did he always put his hand over his mouth when he talked?

3. Youthful Appearance

Youthful appearance is very important in our culture. One of the accepted symbols of this is a bright smile with evenly spaced white teeth.

The loss of an anterior tooth is very destructive to this youthful image; however, the loss of posterior teeth, which "do not show", doesn't evoke the same response in most individuals.

Yet, in truth, the loss of posterior teeth can interfere with chewing and proper diet. This may cause physical ills and accompanying acceleration of ageing. Also, the missing teeth can cause the cheeks to look sunken and old.

4. Social Acceptability

"Sweet smelling breath" is also an important part of being acceptable in our culture. Halitosis (bad breath) can be caused by many factors including dental neglect.

Unfortunately, instead of seeking to correct the cause, the majority of Americans use mouth wash, breath mints and tooth paste to mask the problem and to assure themselves of being "nice to be near". Actually, these are not solutions, they just cover-up the problem.

Mary's classmates thought she was shy, and even sullen, because she rarely smiled or talked. After graduation they were not surprised when she took a job as a file clerk where she rarely talked to anyone and had no contact with the public. Imagine everyone's amazement at the class reunion when a brightly smiling, out-going Mary was telling about her excellent new job dealing with the public.

WHAT MADE THE DIFFERENCE? Mary had been embarrassed by her badly decayed teeth and she was afraid to smile. Her teeth often caused her pain and she felt like a snaggle-toothed witch. After she had her teeth repaired her health was better and she was free of pain. As she learned to smile, her self-esteem improved as did her outlook on life.

AGEING

The loss of teeth, particularly full mouth extractions followed by dentures, holds the very real threat of

> bodily injury,
>
> loss of power, and
>
> a realization of ageing.

These feelings are described here in a fictional monologue by a patient who is about to have new dentures.[4]

The way I look at it, when you start losing your teeth,
you start moving down the other side of the hill;
the more you lose, the faster you go down hill.

If you watch television like me,
you see the same commercials --
the commercials that tell you that good teeth
make you attractive to other people,
particularly the opposite sex.
You know that commercial about sex appeal.

Everytime I plant myself in front of the tube
some good-looking hunk of man or pretty young thing
comes wafting across the screen,
a big, white-teeth smile spreading across
the whole 24 inches of my set.

They do it in a quiet way.
There's no shouting or screaming.
And even if the words aren't just like I hear them,
when I watch the words tell me that it takes sparkling teeth
and sweet-smelling breath to get kissed at least twice.

EXTRACTIONS

<u>MUTILATION</u> is the loss of a
limb or extensive damage to
a part of the body.

Emotionally, one of the greatest
fears the human being faces is
the fear of mutilation.

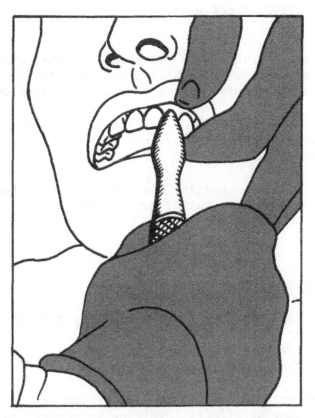

Tooth loss involves a traumatic
intervention, a surgical procedure, and is often viewed, at
least unconsciously, by the patient as a form of mutilation.

Viewed realistically *(when it is
not OUR TOOTH being extracted)* we
expect a rather mild patient reaction when a tooth is extracted.
It has been repeatedly demonstrated
that this is far from the actual
situation.[5]

On a conscious level, we expect the patient to anticipate the procedure in
keeping with the reality of the situation. In actuality, unusual anxieties
and fears are often exhibited by the patient.

There is no doubt of the wide difference between:

> the relatively mild extent
> of the stimuli inherent in
> the extraction viewed externally

and

> the oftentimes intense emotional
> response observed in the dental
> office and operating room.

EXTRACTIONS (continued)

However, it should be stressed here that anxieties and fears connected with the extraction procedures are deeply rooted and spring from fears acquired during the course of the individual's development.

It is not recommended that the dentist (or his staff) probe deeply into the reasons for the fear of loss of a tooth. This would be pointless if not, indeed, unwise.

Still, it is important that the patient's fears be accepted and not ridiculed or put down. No matter how irrational they may seem, these fears are very real to the patient.

THE DENTURE PATIENT

With dentures it is not simply a matter of how they fit, how they look or how they work, but also how the patient uses them, how he puts up with the discomforts involved in adjusting and how he cooperates in the necessary construction procedures.[6]

It is not unreasonable that a person may fear loss of teeth with all of its accompanying effects involving esthetics, masticatory functions and speech.

* Dentures are only 20 to 25 percent as effective as natural teeth.

* The patient will have to learn new ways of talking, chewing, etc.

* The elimination of wrinkles, restoration of fullness to lips and a glamorous smile in a youthful, remolded face (all easily envisioned by the patient) are not likely within the realm of denture service.

* Becoming accustomed to wearing a denture can be a long process that may take months.

The length of time it takes the patient to adjust depends upon the patient and upon the dentist's preparation of this patient both physically and emotionally. Unless the patient is adequately informed in advance of the limitations in function of his complete dentures, he will often complain about their inadequacy.

PRACTICE CYCLE #1

TRUE OR FALSE?

_____1. The fear and anxiety shown by a patient having a tooth extracted are irrational and should be ignored.

_____2. The mouth continues to be psychologically and emotionally important throughout the life of the individual.

_____3. To the patient, the loss of even a single tooth may be viewed as a form of mutilation.

_____4. A properly fitted denture can eliminate all signs of ageing.

_____5. Bad breath can be cured by the use of a good mouthwash.

_____6. Self-image is not adversely affected by decayed or malpositioned teeth.

_____7. The length of time it takes the patient to adjust to dentures depends upon the patient and upon the dentist's preparation of the patient both physically and emotionally.

8. List two ways in which we can benefit from a study of psychology.

_____

_____

_____

9. The_____is the oldest emotionally active part of the body as well as one of the most sensitive.

10. When a baby discovers something new, such as his own foot or a toy, he explores it by_____.

11. The loss of teeth, followed by dentures, holds the very real threat of bodily injury,_____ _____ _____and a realization of_____.

12. List three of the four less commonly recognized ways in which the mouth and teeth are important to the adult.

_____

_____

_____

13. Eruption of the teeth increases the child's power because it:

  (a) Enables him to bite and chew many new _____.

  (b) Increases communication skills as he learns to _____.

  (c) Enables him to express anger and hostility by _____
       and _____ .

14. _____ is damage to the body, usually the loss of a limb,
     or extensive damage to a part of the body.

15. In the adult, aggressive_____ is a socially acceptable form
     of expressing anger and hostility.

FOOD FOR THOUGHT

Mr. Rogers has been forced into what he considers to be an early retirement. Suddenly, he no longer has the prestige and power of his job. He considers himself to be a "has been" and he doesn't like it!

On top of all this, Mr. Rogers' dentist tells him that he has lost his battle against dental disease. Extractions and full dentures are the only solution.

HOW DO YOU THINK MR. ROGERS FEELS ON HEARING THIS?

DO YOU THINK HE WILL BE A DIFFICULT DENTURE PATIENT?

PRACTICE CYLCE #1   FEEDBACK

1. FALSE No matter how irrational these fears may seem, they are very
           real to the patient.

2. TRUE

3. TRUE

4. FALSE A properly fitted denture will greatly improve the patient's
           appearance; however, it cannot be expected to completely eliminate
           signs of ageing.

5. FALSE A mouthwash may mask bad breath; however, it cannot cure it.

6. FALSE Self-image is negatively affected by decayed or malpositioned teeth.

7. TRUE

8. WE CAN BE HELPED TO BETTER UNDERSTAND OURSELVES AND BECOME MORE EFFECTIVE
    IN DEALING WITH OUR OWN PROBLEMS AND IN OUR RELATIONSHIPS WITH OTHERS.

    WE CAN BETTER UNDERSTAND THE PATIENT, BE MORE ACCEPTING OF HIM AS A PERSON,
    AND BE ABLE TO PROVIDE BETTER DENTAL CARE.

9. MOUTH

10. PUTTING IT IN HIS MOUTH

11. LOSS OF POWER   AGEING

12. You could have listed any three of these:

    POWER AND AGGRESSION   YOUTHFUL APPEARANCE

    SELF-IMAGE   SOCIAL ACCEPTABILITY

13. (a) FOODS

    (b) TALK

    (c) BITING AND SPITTING

14. MUTILATION

15. SPEECH

"FOOD FOR THOUGHT" SITUATIONS DO NOT HAVE FEEDBACK.

UNDERSTANDING AND ACCEPTING PATIENT BEHAVIOR

"Mary, what is on the schedule for this morning?" asked Dr. Taylor.

"Oh," replied Mary, "we have an exam, an MOD on a lower first molar, two extractions and a denture adjustment."

This conversation demonstrates how easy it is to forget that our patients are whole human beings -- not just a series of teeth to be treated. This can happen very readily as we concentrate on procedures and techniques; however, understanding, accepting and helping these patients *AS INDIVIDUALS* is an important part of your role as a dental auxiliary.

MOTIVATIONAL FACTORS

The patient is shaped by forces which we cannot see, yet which are vital in determining how the patient will behave and how he will react to the dental situation. These major motivational factors are:

1. SOCIOECONOMIC* BACKGROUND

2. PREVIOUS DENTAL EXPERIENCE

3. REACTION TO THE PRESENT DENTAL SITUATION

4. PSYCHOLOGICAL HEALTH

5. WAYS OF COPING WITH STRESS

*SOCIOECONOMIC is a combination of the words SOCIAL and ECONOMIC. The term refers to all of the ethnic, cultural, family, social and economic factors which make up our background.

MOTIVATIONAL FACTORS (continued)

The following are some of the questions raised by each of the motivational factors. To help us answer these questions, and to better understand the patient and ourselves, we will look at each of these factors in greater depth.

Socioeconomic Background

What attitudes toward dentistry has the patient inherited from his cultural and economic background?

How is he affected by the attitudes of his family and friends?

Previous Dental Experience

Has he received regular care or only emergency treatment?

What has happened during previous treatment which will affect this situation?

Reaction to the Present Dental Situation

How does he feel about his present need for treatment?

Does he feel threatened by it? Does he regard it as a sign of ageing?

Does he fear pain? Does he worry about the expense?

Psychological Health

What are the family, social and economic pressures on him?

What is the present state of his mental health?

Are his actions and reactions normal? neurotic? or psychotic?

Ways of Coping with a Stress Situation

What ways has the patient developed for coping with stress situations?

Are they helpful or do they get in the way of his taking appropriate action?

How can we best help the patient cope with this situation?

OPTIONAL PRACTICE CYCLE

Let's replay that opening dialogue. This time, Dr. Taylor has just asked, "*WHO* is on the schedule for this morning?" Use your imagination and have some fun creating the patients who might be coming in. Tell something about each one. (Obviously there are no right or wrong answers here.)

As an example: *MARK GILES is scheduled for the examination. Mark is three years old, has a lively curiosity (at least that is what his Mother says when he gets into things and takes them apart), and has never been to the dentist before.*

WHO IS COMING FOR THE EXAMINATION? _____

_____

_____

_____

WHO IS SCHEDULED FOR AN MOD ON A LOWER FIRST MOLAR? _____

_____

_____

_____

WHO IS GOING TO HAVE TWO EXTRACTIONS? _____

_____

_____

_____

WHO NEEDS A DENTURE ADJUSTMENT? _____

_____

_____

_____

If you are working with a class, compare notes with your friends. Probably no two of you came up with the same kind of patients for this schedule -- and all answers are right! Dental patients come in all sizes, shapes and varieties. The more you can learn to understand them, the more effective you can be in helping them.

CULTURAL BIAS is the misunderstanding and misinterpretation caused by a member of one class not understanding a member of another class.

Each socioeconomic class within a society has its own customs, standards of living, values, interests and other characteristics which distinguish that class from other socioeconomic levels.

Members of one class generally do not understand the differences between their class and other classes.

Most health workers, including dental auxiliaries, come from the middle class and, therefore, have middle class standards of living, customs, values and standards of behavior.

The middle class worker's expectations regarding patient behavior may be un-realistic for all those patients who are from a different class. We need to be alert to our own tendencies to apply the standards of our socioeconomic class to all patients.

In your work you will come into contact with people from many backgrounds.

*   Some of your patients may come from a different economic background. Some may have known only poverty or economic uncertainty. Others may have had wealth and economic security all their lives.

*   Some may have come from other countries or from homes in which the customs of other nationalities are followed.

*   Some may have been reared in a religious faith with beliefs very different from those you hold.

*   Some may have different educational backgrounds ranging from the Ph.D. to the illiterate.

*   Some may have physical, mental or emotional disabilities.

Your first reaction may be to view these people not only as "different" but also as less acceptable than people who are like you and your friends.

However, it is not your right to judge people, OR to vary the quality of your services because your patient is different in some respect.

CULTURAL BIAS (continued)

The Patient from the Poverty Class

To the middle class, regular dental treatment is an accepted part of living.
To the poor, even emergency care may represent missed meals and one more month
behind on the gas bill!

Poor people have eating habits quite different from middle-class people.
Badly decayed teeth may mean poor diet, lack of knowledge of oral hygiene,
and perhaps ignorance of such things as toothbrushes and flouride toothpastes.

Information about modern health practices is usually unknown to people from
the poverty group. Instead they believe superstitions and "old wives tales"
just as firmly as you believe the information in your textbooks.

To laugh at such beliefs is to indicate a lack of understanding and respect
for others.

The Patient from the Affluent Class

Now let us consider the patient who is from the upper economic level. This
patient does not have financial problems. The necessities of life are assured
because he is able to choose what he wants and pay for it.

However, good health and freedom from pain cannot be assured because of wealth.

It may be difficult for you to understand this patient. He may be critical
and demanding. He may not appear to appreciate what is being done for him.

You may find yourself antagonistic and critical of his actions. It may be
more challenging to provide the services he expects.

Yet,

    he is neither more worthy,

                nor less worthy,

                        than any of your other patients.

THE NEED FOR ACCEPTANCE AND RESPECT

Each of us, no matter what our position in life, has a basic need to be treated with approval and respect. We want others to indicate to us, "You are OK with me and I respect you."

This need becomes greater in times of illness and stress. Although the average dental patient is not ill, he is in a stress situation. Thus, his need for acceptance is great.

We can help the patient by treating him with the same dignity and respect with which we would like to be treated. We can also adopt the philosophy of individual worth.

> *THE PHILOSOPHY OF INDIVIDUAL WORTH is the belief that everyone, regardless of personal circumstances or qualities, has worth. Furthermore, each person is entitled to respect as a human being.*

As a dental auxiliary you will be working with many people. Each one will be different as a person and as a patient.

The challenge is to provide each patient with care which will promote that person's well-being. This requires concern for the patient as an individual, not merely as an upper denture to be fitted or a third molar to be extracted.

Each of your future patients, regardless of socioeconomic status, age, race, religion, or national origin, is a human being with

feelings,

hopes,

problems,

habits,

and needs.

Your greatest challenge is to try to understand these patients in terms of their backgrounds and to try to see situations as they see them.

Applying the Philosophy of Individual Worth

It is easy to give lip service to the philosophy of individual worth. It is quite different to practice it day after day when you have a busy schedule and a wide variety of patients.

However, the degree to which you are successful will influence your effectiveness as a dental auxiliary.

* You may sometimes have difficulty understanding some of your patients, especially those whose cultural background is different from yours.

* You may need to overcome prejudice in order to apply this philosophy to your daily work.

Your responsibility as a dental auxiliary is to know your role, and within that role, to strive to serve EACH of your patients to the best of your ability.

The following suggestions provide a starting point for developing and applying a philosophy of individual worth to your relationships with patients.

1. Learn to accept each patient as an individual with his own unique personality.

2. Recognize that each individual has needs, and is motivated by factors, which are unknown to us.

3. Recognize that each person has his own way of trying to meet his needs. The pattern has developed over his life-time and cannot be changed readily.

4. Make a conscious effort to understand and accept each patient's behavior as he presents himself to you at this point in time.

PRACTICE CYCLE #2

TRUE OR FALSE?

_____1. Each socioeconomic class has its own customs, standards of living and values which distinguish it from other socioeconomic levels.

_____2. Members of one class generally understand and accept the differences between their class and other classes.

_____3. Everyone knows that "old wives tales" are foolish and should be ignored.

_____4. We should treat the patient with the same respect and dignity with which we would like to be treated.

5. Your responsibility as a dental auxiliary is to know your role, and within that role, to strive to serve_____of your patients to the best of your ability.

6. We have a GREATER/LESSER need for approval and respect in times of illness and stress. (Circle correct answer.)

7. _____ _____ is the misunderstanding and misinterpretations caused by a member of one class not understanding a member of another class.

8. The_____ _____ _____ _____ is the belief that everyone, regardless of personal circumstances or personal qualities, has worth.

9. List three motivational factors which may shape patient behavior.

   _____

   _____

   _____

10. These factors WILL/WILL NOT always be known to us. (Circle correct answer.)

11. State two ways in which we can apply the philosophy of individual worth.

   _____

   _____

Please complete the following situations as you think individuals in each group would react.

SITUATION	REACTION		
	POVERTY LEVEL	MIDDLE CLASS	WEALTHY (UPPER CLASS)
A toothache	Trouble! Have tooth pulled as quickly & cheaply as possible.	Treatment (extraction or endodontics) will depend on the state of the budget & other priorities.	Have corrected immediately with the finest treatment available.
Routine dental care	Seek treatment only in case of emergency after all else has failed.	A good idea. It can prevent pain and additional expense.	An accepted part of normal living. A right to which one is entitled.
Preventive dentistry (home care)			
Choice between a silver filling and a gold inlay.			
Loss of all teeth			
Making and keeping dental appointments			

PRACTICE CYCLE #2 FEEDBACK

1. TRUE

2. FALSE Members of one class generally do NOT understand the differences be-
    tween their class and other classes <u>unless</u> they make a conscious
    effort to try to understand.

3. FALSE "Old wives tales" are not foolish to those who believe them. To
    laugh at such tales is to show a lack of respect for the people
    who believe them.

4. TRUE

5. EACH (OR ALL)

6. GREATER

7. CULTURAL BIAS

8. PHILOSOPHY OF INDIVIDUAL WORTH

9. You could have listed any of the following:

    SOCIOECONOMIC BACKGROUND

    PREVIOUS DENTAL EXPERIENCE

    REACTION TO THE PRESENT DENTAL SITUATION

    PSYCHOLOGICAL HEALTH

    WAYS OF COPING WITH STRESS

10. WILL NOT

11. You could have listed any of the following:

    LEARN TO ACCEPT EACH PATIENT

    RECOGNIZE THAT EACH INDIVIDUAL HAS NEEDS

    RECOGNIZE THAT EACH PERSON HAS HIS OWN WAY OF MEETING HIS NEEDS

    MAKE A CONSCIOUS EFFORT TO UNDERSTAND & ACCEPT EACH PATIENT'S BEHAVIOR

There is no feedback for the optional exercise.

PSYCHOTIC, NEUROTIC, OR NORMAL BEHAVIOR?

Human behavior is usually described in terms of being psychotic, neurotic, or normal. However, these are *NOT* clearly delineated categories.

These terms are used to describe *APPROXIMATELY* the level of adequacy of social adjustment which an individual has achieved.

PSYCHOTIC BEHAVIOR

A PSYCHOSIS is a disturbance in thinking or mood which affects the patient's entire personality and behavior.[8]

PSYCHOTIC BEHAVIOR is a behavioral problem so severe and intense, with such deviant reactions, that social adjustment is impossible. Most psychotics require hospitalization for their own protection and for the protection of society.

Examples of psychotic behavior are:

Schizophrenic

In schizophrenic disorders, there is a disorganization of the patient's thought processes. The association of ideas becomes distorted.

Schizophrenic behavior is characterized by disorganization, desocialization, and withdrawal from reality.

Paranoia

In paranoid behavior, there are systematized delusions of grandeur or persecution, or both. These would be characterized by the patient who thinks he is Napoleon or that "they" are out to get him.

Psychopathic

Psychopathic disorders include seriously defective social adjustment, frequently including violent antisocial behavior.

Since these patients usually require hospitalization, they are rarely encountered in the general dental population.

NEUROTIC BEHAVIOR

The NEUROTIC behavioral reaction or disturbance is severe enough that the person can make only a MODERATELY successful social adjustment.

The neurotic can be described as being "maladjusted"; however, these disturbances of behavior are *NOT* so intense that the adjustment is not within the limits we accept in normal social living.

Neurotic disorders represent inadequate and inappropriate methods of dealing with anxiety.

The major difference between psychotic and neurotic behavior is the degree of impairment of social adjustment.

Some of the more common forms of neurotic behavior are:

Anxiety neurosis

This is characterized by emotional tension with apprehension and fearfulness extending to panic.

Depression

This is a state of exaggerated sadness and hopelessness accompanied by reduced activity and a feeling of fatigue without physical cause. The patient feels worthless and has little or no interest in life. Severe depression may require temporary hospitalization.

Hysteria

This is an emotional reaction which is excessive in nature and is characterized by physical symptoms such as fainting.

Hypochondria

A hypochondriac has unreasonable concern about his health. The key words here are "unreasonable concern". This is the patient who always thinks he has something wrong with him, despite medical evidence to the contrary.

Phobias

Phobias are inordinate fears of specific things or situations.

NORMAL BEHAVIOR

The psychotic finds social adjustment impossible,

the neurotic is able to make only a fair social adjustment,

and the so-called normal is able to make a *BETTER THAN FAIR SOCIAL ADJUSTMENT*.

The lines between the normal and neurotic are not clear. An individual may be considered to be normal in most aspects of his behavior and yet be neurotic in others. The average dental patient should be considered to be normal.

The "normal" patient is likely to be:

  * Cooperative during the course of treatment.

  * Report promptly for appointments

  * Carry through on home care

  * And assume his financial obligations as originally arranged.

The normal dental patient will:

  * React to pain, but not show *EXCESSIVE* fear or anxiety.

  * Be relaxed and friendly, yet not too personal, in his relationships with the dentist and his staff.

IT SHOULD BE NOTED HERE

The terms PSYCHOTIC, NEUROTIC and NORMAL are used to describe approximate levels of adequacy of social adjustment which an individual has achieved.

You can use these categories as a frame of reference to recognize patient behavior, to understand it and sometimes to anticipate unusual behavior patterns.

However, it is NOT desirable that you undertake to diagnose or classify the state of the patient's mental health. Referring to patients in these terms is unprofessional and could be slanderous.

PRACTICE CYCLE #3

CASE HISTORIES

MRS. MILLER is not feeling well. She complains that she is always tired, feels sad, and really discouraged about life. She does not care about her appearance, nothing is of interest to her, and she is worried about her health. She has come to the dentist complaining of itching gums and occasional tingling in her teeth. The dentist can find nothing wrong with either Mrs. Miller's teeth or gums.

BARNEY is a college student who has just been through an extensive series of psychological tests. These tests show that he is well adjusted except for his inordinate fear of snakes.

HAROLD loses his temper easily and flies into an uncontrollable rage. When this happens, he grabs a knife, or any handy weapon, and tries to kill whoever is near. Harold is now a patient at the State Mental Hospital.

CYNTHIA is a pretty teenager -- until she smiles and shows her badly decayed teeth. She really wants to have her teeth fixed; however, she is terrified of receiving dental treatment. This fear has prevented Cynthia from receiving the care which she so badly needs and wants.

MARTHA is the mother of two young children. Sometimes she gets tired of changing diapers and listening to baby talk. On the whole, she enjoys family life and her role as a mother. She is healthy, active and enthusiastic in her outlook on life.

1. Is this patient PSYCHOTIC? NEUROTIC? NORMAL? (feel free to add comments).

   Mrs. Miller _____

   Barney _____

   Harold _____

   Cynthia _____

   Martha _____

-25-

PRACTICE CYCLE #3 (continued)

2. Barney's inordinate fear of snakes is called a/an _____.

3. How would you expect this individual to behave as a dental patient?

   Mrs. Miller _____

   _____

   Barney _____

   _____

   Harold _____

   _____

   Cynthia _____

   _____

   Martha _____

   _____

4. A _____ person can make only a moderately successful social adjustment.

5. A _____ requires hospitalization for his own protection and for the protection of society.

6. A person MAY/MAY NOT be neurotic in one area of behavior and normal in other areas. (Circle correct answer.)

7. A "normal" dental patient WILL/WILL NOT show excessive fear or anxiety during treatment. (Circle correct answer.)

8. _____ is excessive emotional reactions characterized by physical symptoms such as fainting.

9. The terms psychotic, neurotic, and normal are used to describe APPROXIMATE/EXACT levels of adequacy of social adjustment which an individual has achieved. (Circle correct answer.)

PRACTICE CYCLE #3 FEEDBACK

1. Mrs. Miller is NEUROTIC. She is depressed as indicated by her constant
    feelings of being tired, sad and not interested in anything. She also
    shows tendencies of being a hypochondriac as indicated by her concern
    about her health and her "unusual" dental symptoms which have no apparent
    cause.

    Barney is NORMAL despite his fear of snakes. Remember we said that a
    person may be considered normal in most aspects of his behavior and yet
    be neurotic in others.

    Harold is PSYCHOTIC. His violent antisocial behavior indicates that he is
    a psychopath.

    Cynthia may be NORMAL or NEUROTIC. Certainly her fear of dentistry would
    be classified as neurotic, particularly to the degree that it prevents
    her from receiving necessary treatment. However, aside from this we do
    not know enough about Cynthia to make a valid judgment.

    Martha is NORMAL. Despite the diapers and baby talk, she seems to be
    enjoying her role in life. She is healthy, active and enthusiastic.

2. Barney has a PHOBIA about snakes.

3. Mrs. Miller will probably be a very difficult dental patient. She is
    apt to come into the office frequently with unusual symptoms which can
    not be dismissed without adequate diagnosis (even if you do suspect she
    is a hypochondriac).

    She is not likely ever to be satisfied with treatment. She may even be
    a "shopper" going from one dental office to the next.

    Because of her depression and accompanying sense of personal worthless-
    ness, she may refuse treatment saying, "No, treatment for the children is
    more important. It is not worthwhile spending money on me."

3. (continued)

<u>Barney</u> should be a normal, cooperative patient.

Since <u>Harold</u> is hospitalized you are not likely to encounter him in the average dental practice. However, if you do, he could very possibly be a model dental patient -- provided he does not become angry!

<u>Cynthia</u> will need a lot of help to even become a dental patient. The **dentist** and his team will have to work with her to help her accept necessary treatment. This will probably require many extra visits.

If her case is severe enough, she may require initial treatment under general anesthesia. Cynthia may also seek other therapeutic aid to help her overcome her fear of dentistry.

<u>Martha</u> is likely to be a normal patient. You may expect her to be co-operative during treatment, to carry through on home care and to meet her finacial obligations. Hopefully, she will also start the children on an early program of preventive dental care.

4. NEUROTIC

5. PSYCHOTIC

6. MAY

7. WILL NOT

8. HYSTERIA

9. APPROXIMATELY

FOR YOUR INFORMATION

ODONTOPHOBIA is an inordinate fear of dental treatment.

PAIN

"Our prime concern as members of the dental profession is control and alleviation of pain. However, in order to control and alleviate pain, we must understand it."[9]

Pain is a protective mechanism. It is a danger signal that says threatening or destructive forces are at work!

PAIN can be defined as suffering or distress of body or mind. It is an unpleasant, uncomfortable response to a stimulus.

The pain stimulus may affect

       any of the five senses

           either singly or in combination,

              or, the stimulus may be only a thought in the mind of an individual.

No matter which, the pain is still very real to the person experiencing it.

Pain is differentiated from other experiences by its unpleasant and unique qualities.

* It is an experience which demands some immediate attention.

* It can become so demanding that it overwhelmes all other senses.

* It disrupts whatever the individual is doing or thinking.

* It drives the individual into some behavior designed to stop the pain as quickly as possible.

PAIN IS A PRIVATE EXPERIENCE

There is no way we can exactly experience the pain of another.
We may have training on which to base our estimate of the patient's pain,
we may be extremely empathetic and understanding;
however, each of us experiences his own pain in his own way.

PAIN THRESHOLD

PAIN THRESHOLD is the point at which the patient becomes aware of the pain.

Pain threshold is approximately the same for everyone regardless of age, cultural background or other variables. It is a constant. That is, a given pain stimulus will produce a pain reaction in most people. However, the way individuals interpret the degree of pain, and react to it, will vary greatly.

PAIN PERCEPTION

PAIN PERCEPTION is the individual's psychological reaction to pain. This is the variable. At the pain threshold, given the same pain stimulus, one person may perceive it as severe pain, another may react to it as mild or moderate pain.

According to Machenzie[10] there are five main variables which affect the psychological perception of pain.

1. Cultural Variables

   Different cultures, and roles within cultures, condition people to respond to pain in a manner consistent with the norms of that culture.

   In a culture where value is placed on stoical forebearance the supresssion of pain expression is expected. In other cultures pain may be expressed openly, even dramatically.

2. Personal History Variables

   The patient's past experience with pain will greatly affect his reaction to any future pain.

   Also personal history factors such as parental attitudes, previous exposure to psychological stress, tension, and even the relationship with the doctor, have been found to influence the perception of pain.

3. Personality Variables

Each individual has generalized patterns and ways of reacting to life. As an example, one person may greet life experiences with the positive outlook of an optimist. Another may be pessimistic and look at all experiences in a negative way.

These life patterns are shaped by many factors including the individual's psychological health. However, the general pattern is applied to most life situations, including the perception of pain.

4. Emotional Variables

There are two ways in which emotion, in the form of anxiety, is related to pain:

   (a) Anxiety intensifies pain and reduces
       tolerance for it.

   (b) Anxiety can actually produce pain.

Also, a tense, anxious patient who is expecting to be hurt will experience a measured amount of pain stimulus to a much more exaggerated degree than a relaxed, confident patient.

5. Cognitive Variables

Knowledge, judgment, concentration and the ability to think are cognitive functions and are useful tools in the control of pain.

The patient who is aware of the source of pain and the reason for it is more accepting of pain than is a patient who isn't informed.

PAIN AND ANXIETY

Although five separate variables have been described, they can be summarized in a single statement,

> *"THE MOST IMPORTANT INFLUENCE ON PAIN*
> *PERCEPTION IS FEAR OR ANXIETY."*

If you look at the five variables you will see that each of them is influenced, or overwhelmed by, fear and anxiety.

According to Joy[11]

> "The level of pain in dentistry today is very low,
>
> but the anxiety level of patients coming into the dental setting is so high that their pain tolerance is extremely low, and they interpret the tiniest stimulus as severe pain."

> *PAINLESS DENTISTRY WILL BECOME A REALITY*
> *WHEN WE HAVE ANXIETY-FREE DENTISTRY !*

Cynthia was finally persuaded to come to the dental office for treatment. However, her fear and anxiety made it impossible for Dr. Taylor to provide even the emergency treatment she needed. She jumped "with pain" almost before even a dental mirror was put in her mouth.

At first, Dr. Taylor used a combination of sedation (to control her anxiety) and local anesthesia (to control the pain) so he could take care of Cynthia's most urgent dental needs.

At succeeding visits, he and his staff worked slowly and patiently with Cynthia until she was able to relax, reduce her level of anxiety, and receive treatment with just local anesthesia.

PRACTICE CYCLE #4

TRUE OR FALSE?

_____ 1. Anxiety can produce pain.

_____ 2. Pain threshold is the point at which the patient becomes aware of pain.

_____ 3. In some cultures, pain may be expressed openly, even dramatically.

_____ 4. The patient's past experience with pain will not affect his reaction to any future pain.

_____ 5. The most important influence on pain perception is fear or anxiety.

_____ 6. It is possible for us to fully understand the pain which the patient is experiencing.

_____ 7. Pain can become so demanding that it overwhelms all other senses.

_____ 8. Pain is a protective mechanism.

_____ 9. Pain threshold is the same in most people; however, pain perception varies greatly.

_____10. The patient who is informed is more accepting of pain than is the patient who isn't informed.

11. The patient's relationship with the doctor WILL/WILL NOT influence his perception of pain. (Circle correct answer.)

12. List three variables which affect pain perception.

_____

_____

_____

PRACTICE CYCLE #4   FEEDBACK

1. TRUE   Anxiety can produce pain. That pain may be entirely mental; however, it is very real to the person experiencing it.

2. TRUE

3. TRUE

4. FALSE The patient's past experience with pain will very definitely affect his future reactions to pain.

5. TRUE

6. FALSE Pain is a very private experience. No matter how well trained or empathetic we may be, we can never fully understand how the other person perceives and reacts to his pain.

7. TRUE

8. TRUE   Pain signals when threatening or destructive forces are at work. These forces do not have to be physical, such as pain from a burn being a warning signal. They may be psychological to warn us that we are in a situation which the mind perceives to be dangerous.

9. TRUE   You and I may experience exactly the same pain, say being stuck with a pin; however, our perception and/or reaction to that pain may be very different.

10. WILL   One reason this is true is because when the patient has a good relationship with the doctor he trusts him. Trust helps reduce anxiety and therefore the perception of pain.

11. You could have listed any of the following:

CULTURAL VARIABLE

PERSONAL HISTORY VARIABLES

PERSONALITY VARIABLES

EMOTIONAL VARIABLES

COGNITIVE VARIABLES

FEAR AND ANXIETY

*"FOR ABOUT 10 MILLION AMERICANS,
FEAR IS THE PRIMARY REASON FOR
FAILURE TO MAKE NECESSARY DENTAL
VISITS."*[12]

FEAR

FEAR is an emotional reaction to a recognized threat.

Fear is the most common emotion in man. It is his preparatory
"flight-or-fight" response to what he perceives as a real danger.

The reaction to fear can be stimulating and constructive IF it helps the
individual avoid threatening or harmful situations.

However, for some, fear is so strong that it paralyzes the individual
so that no action can be taken.

Fear of pain is probably the greatest single contributor to neglected
dental treatment. Inability to afford treatment is very often merely
an excuse.

ANXIETY

*ANXIETY consists of vague feelings arising from threats which cannot be
clearly defined.*

Anxiety is a preparatory flight from a danger that cannot be perceived
or identified by the individual. Anxiety taken to excess can be neurotic
behavior.

The mouth and face are an extremely sensitive zone of the body, highly
charged with emotional significance. Any procedure in or about the mouth
can be expected to arouse anxiety.

FEAR AND ANXIETY TOGETHER

FEAR is flight from the known. ANXIETY is flight from the unknown.

They are often found together. In fact, for the average dental patient it would be difficult, if not impossible, to separate them.

It is not necessary for our understanding of the patient to try to separate and label the difference between fear and anxiety. In fact, we will use the two terms interchangeably.

Is the patient's
distress at the thought
of an injection FEAR? or
ANXIETY?

For many patients it is
a combination of both.

FEAR IS A LEARNED RESPONSE

Fear as a learned response is frequently associated with pain or its anticipation. This type of fear is usually learned by actual experience, such as touching a hot stove.

Children first acquire many of their fears from parents, adults and then from other children. They learn by what they are told and by observing the attitudes and actions of others.

Studies reported by Gale and Ayer[13] indicate two major causes of dental fears:

1. One of the most common causes was anxiety based on the apprehension that the dentist might adopt a negative attitude toward the patient because of neglect of the teeth. *(This relates directly to our need for acceptance and respect.)*

2. The significant difference between fearful and nonfearful dental patients was:

    (a) Unfavorable family dental experience; and

    (b) Unfavorable family attitudes toward dentistry.

According to Dr. Eric Jackson[14], director of a dental fear clinic program, most patients are unaware of the reason for their fear; however, Dr. Jackson and his associates approach the problem as an acquired or learned behavior.

Jack was moderately retarded and, although he was twelve years old, this was his first dental experience. He had been a quiet and cooperative patient most of the time except that he kept asking anxiously, "When you gonna put the silver in?"

When the dentist said to him, "Jack, you've been a good patient and we are almost finished now. All I have to do is put the silver filling in.". At that, Jack started to scream and cry uncontrollably, "No, no, don't do that to me!!!"

Jack was finally calmed enough so he could talk and his story came out. As a joke, one of Jack's relatives told him that the dentist placed a silver filling by pouring hot, melted silver into the tooth. Jack believed this and was terrified of having that hot silver poured into his mouth!

CHILDREN LEARN FEAR FROM ADULTS !

MILD DENTAL FEARS

In the mildest forms, dental fears prevent the patient from cooperating fully in treatment and culminate in:

Lost time for the dentist -- through late arrivals, broken appointments and delaying tactics.

Unnecessary difficulty in performing dental procedures -- often requiring special procedures and additional chairtime.

And frequently unsatisfactory end-results -- because of the patient's inability to cooperate, the dentist may not be able to provide optimal dental treatment.

EXTREME DENTAL FEARS

For those with intense dental fear the mere thought of dental care is extremely anxiety-provoking. Consequently treatment, even in the presence of severe pain, is avoided.

The resulting poor oral health may affect the patient in the following ways:

* Loss of teeth and periodontal disease because of poor oral hygiene and lack of dental care.

* Poor nutrition because of the inability to eat properly due to the loss of teeth, breakdown of teeth, and/or pain in the mouth. This can lead to systemic diseases.

* Poor general health because infection and disease in the mouth can spread throughout the body. These also weaken the body's resistance to other diseases.

* Psychological ill-health because of pain, unattractive appearance and insecurity about bad breath and youthful appearance.

FEAR AND ANXIETY EXPRESSED

Fear and anxiety can be manifested physically, psychologically and emotionally. Often they appear in a form which is difficult to recognize for what it is.

Physical Signs of Fear

* Tense face and white-knuckle gripping of the chair arm.

* Profuse perspiration even in a cool room.

* Trembling and shallow breathing.

* Changes in pulse rate, blood pressure and respiration.

* Fainting.

Psychological and Emotional Manifestations (plus many others)

* Seeming distraction, preoccupation and social withdrawal.

* Inappropriate elation and cheerfulness.

* Unsolicited denial of fear and no overt show of fear or anxiety.

* Denial of the situation, constant turning of attention elsewhere.

* Quarrelsomeness and disruptive behavior.

* Seeming resentment toward those who are trying to relieve his pain.

* Hostility and responses inappropriate to the situation.

"Perhaps the most important single tool we can use is an ATTITUDE which regards this fear of dental treatment and its expression as part of the problem we are called upon to deal with -- rather than an annoying obstacle which stands in the way of our proper function."

Borland[15]

PRACTICE CYCLE #5

1. State Trooper Dawson marched into the operatory, somewhat casually slung his gun belt over the back of a chair, sat down and FAINTED!

   Since he is in good health, except for a persistent toothache, what do you think caused him to faint? _____

   _____

   _____

2. When we talked about pain we mentioned that our culture places certain expectations on us as to how we will express our reaction to pain or fear.

   Do you think it would have been "culturally acceptable" for Trooper Dawson to come into the dental office trembling and talking about how afraid he was of the dentist? _____

   _____

3. Any procedure in or about the mouth CAN/CANNOT be expected to arouse anxiety. (Circle correct answer.)

4. One of the two major causes of dental fear was listed as "anxiety based on the apprehension that the dentist might adopt a negative attitude because of neglect of the teeth."

   Please state this in your own words. _____

   _____

   _____

5. Do you think the above is true for many patients? _____
   Would it be true for you? _____
   How do you think this attitude would affect planning and carrying out a preventive dentistry and home care program? _____

   _____

   _____

6. We quoted Borland talking about attitude being an important tool in our response to the patient's fear. State in your own words how you feel this relates to our acceptance of the patient as a whole person, not just teeth to be treated. _____

_____

_____

_____

7. Mother had a dental appointment. She spent days telling everyone how much she dreaded it and came home afterward moaning about how awful it was. Although nothing was said directly to little Susie, how do you think this will affect her future attitude toward going to the dentist?

_____

_____

8. When it comes time for Susie's first dental appointment, do you think she will believe her mother when she says, "There is nothing to it. You will like that nice Dr. Taylor. He won't hurt you."? _____

_____

9. _____ is an emotional response to a recognized threat.

_____ is a response to threats that cannot be clearly defined or identified.

10. We quoted Jackson as saying that most patients are not aware of the reason for their dental fears. Why do you think this is so?

_____

_____

_____

_____

_____

PRACTICE CYCLE #5 FEEDBACK
_____

1. Trooper Dawson's fainting was probably a physical manifestation of his
    FEAR AND/OR ANXIETY.

2. This is a matter of opinion. I doubt that he would consider it "culturally
    acceptable". Hopefully, as we move away from stereotyped roles such as the
    male having to be big and strong, people like the trooper will feel free
    to express their anxiety in more direct ways.

3. CAN The mouth is extremely important to us in many, many ways. Anything
         that threatens the mouth can be counted on to arouse anxiety.

4. You might have stated something to the effect that, "When the patient
    goes to the dentist he knows that the dentist is in a real power position
    and he doesn't want to do anything to displease him. The patient is also
    aware that caring for teeth is very important to the dentist. The patient
    may be afraid that the dentist will reject, or dislike, him because he has
    not taken care of his teeth."

5. YES or NO is an acceptable answer. Again, this is a matter of opinion.
    It is probably true for most patients than we would expect. This is
    one of those vague fears that is not easily expressed.

    YES or NO (whichever is true for you.)

    This attitude can be very important in planning a preventive dentistry
    program. Here the dentist, and his auxiliaries, are placing responsibility
    with the patient for the preventive care of his teeth.

    If the patient doesn't follow through he may feel that he has failed in
    his responsibility and he may once again be fearful that the dentist
    won't like him because he hasn't done what he was told.

6. You might have stated something like this, "An anxious patient may slow
    treatment and cause us extra work. However, when we accept him as a whole
    person we must also accept his fears and anxieties. Hopefully, we will
    be able to help this patient overcome these problems."

7. Mother's actions will most certainly affect little Susie's future attitude toward the dentist. As we said, children learn their fears from their parents and adults, and then from other children. Many of these fears are learned from observing what the big people do -- not necessarily what they say.

8. When it comes time for Susie to go to the dentist there is no way she is going to believe all those nice things Mother is telling her about Dr. Taylor. The seeds of fear have already been sown, and more were added when Mother introduced the idea of pain with her statement, "He won't hurt you." (Up to now Susie didn't know it was supposed to hurt.) Despite the fact that Susie has never been to the dentist before, Dr. Taylor may have to treat a very apprehensive patient.

9. FEAR

    ANXIETY

10. This, too, is a matter of opinion and there are many reasons you could give. Some of them are the following:

    We develop our fears and anxieties gradually over a lifetime. Rarely is there a single trigger-event which we can identify as the one causative factor.

    We have a marvelous protective mechanism by which we tend to forget our unpleasant experiences. Although these are out of our conscious awareness, they are stored in our unconscious. Therefore, although we are no longer consciously aware of them, these early experiences still influence our behavior and reactions.

    Adverse attitudes toward dentistry come from many factors outside of our awareness. Cartoons and television programs which depict the dentist in a negative way may influence us, just as the attitudes of our family and friends will.

STRESS

Medical and psychological problems caused by stress have become the NUMBER-ONE HEALTH PROBLEM of the last decade.[16]

FLIGHT, FIGHT OR SUBMIT

STRESS can be defined as any factor which causes physical or emotional tension.

Stress producing factors, whether physical or emotional, stimulate the body in a flight-or-fight response. The instant the brain receives the stress alarm, it alerts the body to prepare for vigorous exertion. This reaction is ideal to ward off physical danger, but can cause serious consequences when there is no one to fight, no place to run.

Our culture has added a third element to the primitive flight-or-fight response. That is, SUBMIT. There are many situations in which we can neither fight nor flee. Despite our stress we must stay and cope.

Also, we are continually faced with increasing numbers of long term stress situations. These may be caused by our family and other relationships, work and/or our environment.

All of life is composed of widely varying levels and kinds of stress. Stress in itself is neither good nor bad. Happy occasions, like marriage or the birth of a child, cause stress. So do negative events such as pain, fear or anxiety.

The dental patient is in a temporary stress situation because of his reaction to receiving treatment. His gut level response may be flight-or-fight, yet he knows he must stay and submit.

Just as important are the outside stress factors which the patient brings with him from other aspects of his life. Unfortunately, these are usually unknown to the dentist and his staff.

Marion Welsh is usually a pleasant and cooperative patient. However, today she seems on the verge of tears and jumps everytime Dr. Taylor picks up the handpiece. What the doctor doesn't know, at least until he stops and asks if anything is wrong, is that Marion's youngest child is ill with what may be rheumatic fever. Also, she has just gotten word that her husband must accept a transfer or lose his job. Marion's stress has nothing to do with her dental treatment -- yet it does affect her behavior as a patient.

STRESS IMPROPERLY HANDLED BECOMES DISTRESS

Stress is a well-documented cause of

    anxiety,

        depression,

            migraine headache,

                ulcers,

                    heart disease,

                        and stroke.

Research is underway to determine if stress may cause periodontal disease.

Most of the body's reactions to stress are normal and appropriate. After a person meets a specific challenge, his body returns to its normal level of activity relatively quickly. However, stress becomes pathological when the body reacts as though it is threatened long after the actual threat has passed.

The effect of stress is determined not by the stress itself, but by how we view and react to that stress. Also, stress is subjective. The degree of stress that is tolerable to one person may be unbearable to the next.

Whatever the level or type of stress, man reacts to it by seeking to adjust. He does this by applying the various resources which are available to him. Serious problems arise only when stress is so severe that the individual is unable to muster sufficient resources to overcome it.

FOR YOUR INFORMATION

Some people, in long term stress and tension producing situations, may clench their teeth or develop bruxism. (BRUXISM is the habitual grinding and gritting of the teeth.) This most frequently occurs when the patient is asleep and he is often unaware of what he is doing. These habits may cause excessive wear of the teeth, severe periodontal problems including bone loss, and temporomandibular joint problems.

To prevent further damage to the teeth and surrounding tissues, the dentist may make a night guard mouth protector to be worn by the patient when he is asleep.

COPING WITH STRESS

DEFENSE MECHANISMS are the individual's way of actively coping with a threathening, stress producing, situation.

Of necessity, we have all developed ways of helping ourselves cope with stress situations and some of the things we do are called defense mechanisms. Many of these are on a subconscious level and may be carried out without our being aware of them.

Defense mechanisms can be useful coping behavior; however, they become neurotic and destructive when they interfere with action which could stave off the danger.

As an example - the individual who keeps forgetting to make, or keep, his dental appointments until it is too late to save his teeth has carried his defense mechanism so far that it has become neurotic behavior.

On the other hand - the patient who uses his defense mechanisms to enable him to cope with his stress about the dental situation, thereby being able to receive appropriate treatment, is using his defense mechanisms in a positive and beneficial manner.

Let's look at some of the most commonly used defense mechanisms.

Repression

Repression is the selective forgetting of things that are tension producing in the individual. Often this is done on a subconscious level. It may be described as the individual philosophy of "If I ignore it, it will go away!" An example of this is the patient who repeatedly "forgets" to make or keep his dental appointments.

THE ICEBERG PRINCIPLE[17]

It is estimated that a floating iceberg is only one-tenth visible. Nine-tenths of the ice block remains submerged beneath the surface of the water. A similar estimate has been suggested with regard to human emotions. The part that we are able to see is only about one-tenth of the total reality. The implication of this suggestion is not that people show only one-tenth of their true recognized feelings to others, but rather that they are consciously aware of only a small part of their own emotions. We hide the bulk of our emotions even from ourselves by the subconscious defense mechanism called repression.

COPING WITH STRESS (continued)

Deployment

Deployment is the process of getting your mind off what is going on.
It is a powerful and effective means of coping unless it prevents necessary action.

In using deployment of attention away from the threat, the patient dis-
tracts himself. He focuses his attention on his mother-in-law, on his
goldfish, on his income tax return -- anywhere but on his mouth.

Control

When we have control of a situation we have the power to regulate and
direct what is happening.

Control is a key factor in coping with stress, yet individual responses
vary greatly. Some people are most comfortable sitting back passively
and handing control over to others. Some people feel comfortable only
so long as they control their fate, only as long as they have a hand in
determining what happens next.[18]

The patient does not have much feeling of being in control of the
situation when he is supine in the dental chair with two pairs of
hands and assorted instruments in his mouth, and various hoses draped
across his chest.

Borland[19] reports that many patients have remarked about the intolerable
lack of control which they feel during such procedures.

In fact, much dental treatment is an outstanding example of a situation in
which the patient must not only submit to a procedure which he fears, he
must also turn most of the control over to others.

We say most of the control because there are many ways in which the patient
retains some control. Among these are: coming late for his appointment,
excessive questions which delay treatment, frequent requests to rest or spit,
even the manner in which he pays his bill.

When the patient feels he can trust the dentist and his team, then it is
easier for him to relinquish control of the situation.

COPING WITH STRESS (continued)

Regression

Regression is retreat to an earlier, less mature, level of adjustment.

When we are ill, or in a stress situation, we may temporarily regress. That is, we may return to an earlier level of behavior which had previously been comfortable for us.

This is often seen in children.

* They may cry when they've outgrown the crying stage.

* They may revert to baby talk or nonverbal communication such as crying, kicking and screaming, when they are quite adept with verbal language.

* They may cling to their mother despite the fact that most of the time they are very independent.

* They may go back to thumb sucking when this habit has been stopped.

Adults do it, too!

* They may become more demanding and childish.

* They may become self-centered and apparently unaware of the rights and needs of others.

* The "former smoker" may go back to smoking.

* The "former drinker" may go back to drinking.

FOR YOUR INFORMATION

ANGER is a secondary emotion which is generated by an individual's inability to make a more appropriate response to stress, fear or anxiety.

HOSTILITY is the acting-out of anger.

Affiliation

When we face trouble we seek the company of someone we know and trust. Danger never seems as threatening if we meet it in the presence of familiar faces.

The dental patient wants to feel that he is among friends who care. He wants to know that those who are treating him are professionally competent and genuinely concerned about his well-being. He wants to be able to trust them.

A seven-year old child described it well for all of us when he said,

> *"I hope you know what you're doing, because it's ME
> and I don't want anything to happen to me!"*[20]

YOU ARE NOT THE TARGET ! ! !

We've talked about a lot of factors which influence the patient's behavior and the ways in which he may respond to these stresses.

It is important for you to realize that the patient is not necessarily reacting to you as an individual.

He is acting out his own needs, his own situation, and using his own ways of coping.

Although his behavior may seem to be aimed at you --

YOU ARE NOT THE TARGET!

You will be happier, more effective in your work, and reduce your own level of stress, when you are able to keep the situation in perspective.

You should try to accept the patient as you find him, and not feel threatened or react negatively to his seemingly hostile behavior.

PRACTICE CYCLE #6

MATCHING

_____ 1. REPRESSION

_____ 2. DEFENSE MECHANISMS

_____ 3. DEPLOYMENT

_____ 4. CONTROL

_____ 5. REGRESSION

(a) Retreat to an earlier, less mature
     level of adjustment.

(b) The process of getting your mind
     off what is going on.

(c) When in danger we seek the company
     of someone we know and trust.

(d) The selective forgetting of things
     that are tension producing in the
     individual.

(e) The individual's way of actively
     coping with a threatening, stress
     producing situation.

(f) The power to regulate and direct
     what is happening.

TRUE OR FALSE?

_____ 6. All stress is harmful.

_____ 7. Stress-caused disorders are the number-one health problem
            of the last decade.

_____ 8. The degree of stress that is tolerable to one person
            may be unbearable to the next.

_____ 9. The third element added to the flight-or-fight response is stress.

_____ 10. Defense mechanisms may be harmful if they prevent necessary
            action.

PRACTICE CYCLE #6 (continued)

TRUE OR FALSE? (continued)

_____11.   According to the "Iceberg Principle" we hide the bulk of our emotions
             even from ourselves by the defense mechanism called regression.

_____12.   When the patient seems negative or hostile, you are not necessarily
             the target or the cause of his attitudes and actions.

PRACTICE CYCLE #6   FEEDBACK

1.   D

2.   E

3.   B   (c) is AFFILIATION

4.   F

5.   A

6.   FALSE   Stress is a protective mechanism.   It is our response to stress
             that can be harmful.

7.   TRUE

8.   TRUE

9.   FALSE   Stress causes the flight-or-fight response.   The third element
             added by our culture is SUBMIT.

10. TRUE

11. FALSE   We hide things from ourselves by REPRESSION.   Regression is
             going back to a less mature level of behavior.

12. TRUE

SECTION TWO: HELPING THE DENTAL PATIENT

TRUST BUILDING

THE PATIENT WANTS TO KNOW THAT HE HAS COME TO THE RIGHT PLACE!

Perhaps the single most important element in the dentist/staff-patient relationship is trust.

When the patient trusts those treating him he will:

* Be more accepting of their professional judgment.

* Be more relaxed, less anxious and better able to cooperate in his own treatment.

* Be more comfortable in turning control of the situation over to those caring for him.

Trust building is a gradual process which cannot be rushed. It begins with the patient's first contact with the dental office and continues throughout the professional relationship.

There are many factors which affect trust building and many ways in which the dental health team members can help this process happen.

LET'S BE FRIENDS

We trust friends more than we do strangers. And when we are in a stress situation we want to know that we are among friends.

The following are some of the ways in which you can help the patient feel that he is with people who care and are his friends.

1. Wear a name tag and introduce yourself to new patients.

2. Call the patient by name. This makes the patient feel better and enables you to be sure you have the right patient and the right chart. However, do not call the patient by his first name unless you are certain that this is acceptable to him.

3. Be considerate of the patient as an individual. Take a personal interest and make an effort to remember information about family, hobbies, or special events that seem to be of interest. (Putting a note in the chart will help remind both you and the doctor.)

AS THE PATIENT SEES US

First impressions are critical in the development of a good relationship with the patient. The patient's impression of the office begins with his first contact when he telephones for an appointment. They form ever more rapidly when he actually arrives at the office for the first time.

The Telephone

> *Patients want the telephone voice on the other end to be concerned, accepting of them and their feelings, and warm and friendly -- rather than cold, distant and businesslike.*

The receptionist answering the telephone has the first opportunity to let the patient know that this is an office with a staff that cares about people, not just teeth!

The telephone should be answered promptly and pleasantly by identifying both the office and the speaker. As an example, "Good morning, Dr. Taylor's office. Mary Wells speaking."

The conversation should be warm and friendly, yet businesslike. It is possible to convey caring without carrying on a long personal conversation.

Greeting the Patient

The patient's arrival should be treated as a pleasant event -- not an unwelcome interruption of more important routine!

He should be greeted warmly, promptly and by name. If possible, give the patient a realistic estimate of how long he will have to wait. (This lets the patient know that we respect him by respecting his time.)

Returning patients appreciate some indication that they are remembered and that you are happy to see them again.

New patients want reassurance that they are welcome here and that they will be treated with consideration.

Visible Cleanliness

Visible cleanliness is extremely important for it is often the layman's yardstick for judging the competence of professional care.

The reception room is a key location, for it is here that the patient forms one of his first impressions of the dentist, his office and staff. All this happens long before any actual dental treatment has been provided.

We can help by:

Seeing that ash trays are emptied regularly (if smoking is permitted) and that the area is aired regularly.

Keeping toys in their area and out of pathways where people walk. Toys say welcome to children; however, if they are allowed to be messy they are both hazardous and uninviting to others.

Being sure reading materials are in good condition, appropriate and relatively recent.

Occasionally taking time to go into the reception room and looking at it critically as the new patient does.

The patient must accept on trust that appropriate sterilization and disinfection methods are being used. He can judge the sanitary standards of the office only by what he sees.

He can see when the operatory is obviously neat and clean.

He can see when the auxiliary washes her hands each time she returns to the chair.

He can see spots on a uniform. In his imagination, the patient may envision these as blood from an unfortunate previous patient -- or as catsup stains left over from the assistant's prior job as a waitress. Neither of these flights-of-fancy does anything to build the patient's level of trust and confidence!

PROFESSIONAL COMPETENCE

The level of professional competence of his staff reflects directly on
the dentist. Often the patient will perceive the dentist as being no
more, or less, competent than the people he selects to work with him.

Self-Respect

An important part of professional competence is self-respect. An auxiliary
who knows she is capable is able to go about her duties calmly and effectively, yet remain fully human. She doesn't have to hide behind a starchy
cold mask of efficiency.

In the eyes of the patient, appearance is an important part of professional
competence. No matter how relaxed the dress code or uniform regulations
are in your office, you should always appear neat, well groomed and clean.
The patient may well equate sloppy appearance with sloppy performance and
the patient wants your BEST performance when you are caring for him.

Calm

Calm is a key word in describing professional competence.

The patient very quickly senses the emotional atmosphere of the office.
He picks up on any tension and this adds to his own stress level.

In case of an emergency the patient's reaction, to a large degree, depends
upon that of those caring for him.

If everyone becomes excited and is frantically running around, the patient
will become alarmed. On the other hand, if personnel respond to the situation in a calm, "everything is under control" manner, the patient will
be reassured.

> Know your role in emergency procedures. Practice until
> you are sure you can perform calmly in a stress situation.

> Select your words and monitor your tone of voice carefully.
> This is a situation in which what-you-say AND how-you-say-it
> are both important.

STAFF ATTITUDES

The dentist and his staff who have a warm relationship communicate this kind of supportive and caring attitude to the patient.

When the staff obviously like, trust and respect the dentist (and each other), the patient quickly senses this. It helps him develop his own trust level.

Warmth, respect and empathy are three major factors in conveying to the patient that we are concerned about him as a person and that he can trust us.

Warmth

Warmth is communicating, verbally and nonverbally, to the patient that you care about him and his situation. We transmit this warmth by our tone of voice, a reassuring touch, considerate attitude and sincere interest in the patient.

Patients very quickly detect when we are being insincere and phoney in our approach to them.

Respect

Respect is the positive acknowledgment, verbally and nonverbally, of the unique personhood of the patient.

We identified in Section One that the need for respect is important in all of us, particularly in times of stress. The most effective way to convey respect to the patient is to treat him with the dignity we desire for ourselves.

Acceptance is an important aspect of respect. One study we quoted reported that patients were afraid to go to the dentist for fear that he would not like (accept) them because they had neglected their teeth. Our obvious acceptance of the patient (as we find him, not as we wish him to be), will help allay that patient's fear of rejection.

Verbal and nonverbal signals make up the two parts of every communication between people. Verbal signals are the words we use. Nonverbal signals, often called body language, consist of facial expression, tone of voice, and the way we hold our body, move, sit and act.

Empathy

Empathy is knowing and communicating to the patient that you realize how he feels. It does not in any way criticize these feelings -- even when you may believe the feelings to be wrong.

Empathy means understanding feelings, but *DOES NOT MEAN SHARING THE OTHER'S FEELINGS*. For example, if you are attempting to help a person who is anxious and you begin to feel anxious, that is NOT being empathic.

> Self-understanding and other-understanding seem to exist as two sides of the same coin of empathy. The ability to understand another person seems to be dependent, at least to some degree, on the ability to understand and accept yourself.
>
> You don't have to completely understand yourself before you can understand another. Rather, this growth seems to happen at the same time and is mutually supportive. That is, the more you understand and accept yourself, the better you are able to understand and accept others as they are.[21]

One of the basic requirements for developing empathic understanding is that you pay attention to the expressions of the patient. Paying attention means that your senses are alert to the behavior of the patient.

That is you LOOK AT and LISTEN TO the patient.

Looking at a person provides massive information including nonverbal clues such as gestures, facial expressions, body position, muscle tone, skin coloration, eye movement, etc.

Listening to a person provides the insight to a better understanding of interests, experiences, problems and concerns.

If you are really concentrating on understanding him

the patient will usually tell you, verbally and/or nonverbally,

when you are understanding or when you are misunderstanding.

A SENSE OF HUMOR

The professional office does not have to be cold and unfriendly in its atmosphere. Everyone involved is very human and this is best reflected in a well directed sense of humor. Laughing together helps develop a sense of warmth and closeness.

However, there are several precautions to be observed here.

1. Practical jokes and off-color humor are out of place. Never tell a joke or make any remark you would not make to your prudish Aunt Matilda. You don't know how the patient feels about these things and you should not take chances. (This includes discussing politics.)

2. Don't laugh or joke where the patient may hear you but is not included. He may well assume that you are laughing at him. Include the patient in the fun. He probably needs a good laugh.

   On the other hand, be sensitive. If the patient is really upset, nothing is amusing to him and you don't want him to feel that you are making light of his concerns.

3. Never make the patient the butt of a joke or any comment which could make him uncomfortable. Since we can't know all of the patient's background, extreme caution is advised.

4. Don't let joking and kidding interfere with patient care! The patient wants to know you are paying strict and serious attention to his treatment. Bantering between doctor and auxiliary may be fun but you should be aware of how the patient may interpret it.

5. Funny patient stories can be a riot but NOT to another patient! If you laugh about one patient, this one may think that you will laugh about him, too.

   Also, remember that you must respect the confidentiality of patient information. This means you can't tell that funny story at the bridge table either. (RECOMMENDED READING: *Ethics and Jurisprudence.*)

PRACTICE CYCLE #7

1. We convey to the patient that we care about him as a person through our attitudes of _____ , _____ and _____ .

2. The single most important element in the dentist/staff-patient relationship is _____ .

3. _____ is knowing and communicating to the patient that you realize what he is feeling.

4. _____ _____ is often the layman's yardstick for judging the competence of professional care.

5. In developing empathic understanding we need to _____ _____ and _____ _____ the patient.

6. New patients DO/DO NOT want reassurance that they are welcome here and that they will be treated with consideration. (Circle correct answer.)

7. List at least one way in which we convey our professional competence (or lack of it) to the patient.

   _____

   _____

8. List two factors which are important in trust building.

   _____

   _____

   _____

9. List at least one way in which we convey warmth to the patient.

   _____

   _____

TRUE OR FALSE?

_____10. The patient forms his first impression of the dental office
            after he has received treatment.

_____11. Patients often perceive the dentist as being no more, or no
            less, competent than the people he selects to work with him.

_____12. To show warmth, a telephone conversation must be long and personal.

_____13. A sense of humor is always out of place in a professional office.

_____14. The patient who trusts those caring for him will be more com-
            fortable in turning control of the situation over to them.

_____15. In the professional office, both what-you-say and how-you-say-it
            are important.

John! Mary!

You may want to try the old drama school exercise which is used to teach
actors to express emotion through just the tone of voice.

There are two characters, each with one word of dialog. John's word is,
'Mary." Mary's word is, "John."

Working with a friend, with one of you playing John and the other being
Mary, use just the two words of dialog and express the following feelings:

| GREETING | SURPRISE | LOVE | ANGER |

| SADNESS | FEAR | PARTING |

PRACTICE CYCLE #7   FEEDBACK

1. WARMTH, RESPECT, EMPATHY

2. TRUST

3. EMPATHY

4. VISIBLE CLEANLINESS

5. LOOK AT   LISTEN TO

6. DO

7. SELF-RESPECT or a CALM ATTITUDE could have been listed.
    (There are also many other "right" answers as to how we convey
    professional competence.)

8. You could have listed any two of the following:

    BEING FRIENDLY & GENUINELY CONCERNED

    CREATING A FAVORABLE IMPRESSION

    POSITIVE STAFF ATTITUDES AND TREATING PATIENTS WITH WARMTH, RESPECT & EMPATHY

    CONVEYING PROFESSIONAL COMPETENCE

9. You could have listed any of the following: TONE OF VOICE,

    REASSURING TOUCH, CONSIDERATE ATTITUDE, SINCERE INTEREST.

10. FALSE First impressions are formed long before any treatment
           has been rendered.

11. TRUE

12. FALSE A conversation can convey warmth without being long or personal.

13. FALSE A well directed sense of humor is a great asset in a professional
           office.

14. TRUE

15. TRUE

HAVE YOU EVER BEEN IN THIS KIND OF SITUATION?	WHAT DO YOU REMEMBER MOST VIVIDLY? HOW DID YOU FEEL?
You arrive on time for your appointment. You wait 15 minutes and still no one has acknowledged your arrival.	
You telephone a professional office. Someone answers the phone by saying, "hold please" and then disappears from the line without giving you a chance to say anything.	
In an office where you are a new patient you notice stains on the floor, finger prints on the walls, and spots on the auxiliary's uniform. The whole place looks slightly out-dated, sloppy and messy.	
The auxiliary who is about to take study models on you has cigarette stains on her fingers, onions on her breath and hair that falls in her face so that she has to keep using her hand to push it back.	
You dial your doctor's office. Someone answers the telephone just saying "hello." You don't know if you have reached the right number.	

RESPONSIVE LISTENING

THERE ARE MANY WAYS TO RESPOND TO THE PATIENT.

> *SOME ARE HELPFUL,*
>
> > *SOME ARE HARMFUL,*
> >
> > > *OTHERS ARE AT BEST NEUTRAL.*

The dental auxiliary needs to learn to be a good listener and be able to respond effectively to the message sent by the patient.

Good listening requires that you concentrate totally on the patient.

* You do not let your mind wander. You put aside personal concerns while the patient is talking.

* You are not busy formulating your reply or rushing ahead to what you feel is a good conclusion.

* You are listening and looking. This way you can pick up both the verbal and nonverbal information the patient is transmitting.

Being responsive to the patient takes listening one step further. It requires being sensitive to what the patient is expressing in terms of feelings and needs.

The same way of responding is not appropriate to all situations. It is important that you learn how to listen carefully and respond appropriately.

One patient may want to get his mind off the situation by discussing the weather or a good book he has read.

Another may want an opportunity to express and explore his feelings about the situation.

Being responsive must start with leaving control of the conversation with the patient. It is inappropriate for the auxiliary to try to force the patient into expressing feelings when this is not what he wants.

An effective responsive listener lets the patient take the conversational lead, remains sensitive to when he wants to change topics, and is alert to clues that he wishes to terminate the conversation.

RESPONSES THAT DO NOT HELP

Irrelevant Statement

An irrelevant statement is a response which is not at all related to the patient's expressed feelings.

> PATIENT: *"I was so nervous about coming today that I couldn't eat my breakfast."*

> IRRELEVANT RESPONSE: *"Oh, what do you usually have for breakfast?"*

Such a response lets the patient know that you did not really hear the fear he was trying to express and he may feel that you are not sincerely interested in him.

"Hitch-hiking" is another form of irrelevant response. In this you listen, just waiting for the patient to say something that you can pick up on and take off on your own train of thought.

> PATIENT: *"I've been having trouble getting my little boy to brush his teeth."*

> HITCH-HIKING RESPONSE: *"You think that is trouble! Why, my little sister etc., etc., etc."*

An Evaluative Statement

An evaluative statement is one which tells that patient that you do NOT approve of his feelings.

> PATIENT: *"I hate going to the dentist. I am afraid of the pain."*

> EVALUATIVE RESPONSE: *"That is a lot of foolishness! Modern dentistry is almost painless and there is nothing to fear."*

This leaves the patient feeling put-down and discounted. With such an answer he is certainly not going to feel respected or accepted.

RESPONSES THAT ARE NEUTRAL

A Supportive Response

A supportive response tells the patient that it is acceptable to feel the way he does and offers him support. It is the type of statement used most frequently by health professionals.

> PATIENT: *"I am really worried about this extraction."*
>
> SUPPORTIVE RESPONSE: *"No need to be, it does not seem to be a very difficult one. It should not take more than about ten minutes."*

The supportive statement has limitations in its effectiveness. It tends to put an end to the discussion and it does not encourage the patient to go further in expressing his feelings.

However, it is a very appropriate response for use by the auxiliary. Unless your doctor has encouraged you to help the patients express their feelings, and unless you feel qualified to do this, you may be most comfortable with this level of response.

RESPONSES THAT HELP

Reflective Listening

Reflective listening communicates to the patient that he is being listened to and understood. It involves hearing his meaning and feelings accurately, and then reflecting this back to the patient in other words.

> PATIENT: *"Must I have a needle?"*
>
> RELECTIVE RESPONSE: *"You are afraid that the injection will hurt."*

In reflective listening you say the same thing in a different way, with different words, to reflect how you perceive the speaker is feeling.

This provides the speaker with feedback that you are indeed listening carefully to him and understanding what he is expressing. If what you have reflected is incorrect, he will soon let you know.

RESPONSES THAT HELP (continued)

Reflective Listening (continued)

As you learn to be a reflective listener you become increasingly sensitive to:

1. The words the speaker is saying and how he is saying them.

2. The feelings implied by his words.

3. His facial expression and use of body language.

At first, reflective listening seems strange and artificial -- almost as if you're being a parrot. However, with practice it becomes easier and more natural. Also, with experience you are able to reflect the deeper feelings which the patient may not be able to express clearly even to himself.

Reflective listening, coupled with a warm and willing silence, leaves the patient in control of the situation. If he wants to say more he will feel free to do so. Or, you may use door-opener expressions such as, "I see", "Oh" or "Would you like to talk about it?" The important thing to remember is that you must not push the patient into an unwanted or inappropriate exploration of feelings.

ROADBLOCKS TO COMMUNICATION

Reflective listening can be an affective problem solving tool to use when the other person has the problem and you are willing to help him try to solve it for himself. Reflective listening leaves control and responsibility with the person who owns the problem. (This technique is not appropriate to use when you have a mutual or shared problem.)

Thomas Gordon, in his book Parent Effectiveness Training[22], lists twelve road-blocks to communication. These blocks, listed on the next page, stop communication when you use them, instead of trying to help someone through responsive listening.

THE TWELVE ROADBLOCKS TO COMMUNICATION

1. ORDERING, DIRECTING, COMMANDING
   Telling the person to do something, giving him an order or a command.

2. WARNING, ADMONISHING, THREATENING
   Telling the person what consequences will occur if he does something.

3. EXHORTING, MORALIZING, PREACHING
   Telling the person what she should or ought to do.

4. ADVISING, GIVING SOLUTIONS OR SUGGESTIONS
   Telling the person how to solve a problem, giving her advice or
   suggestions; providing answers or solutions for her.

5. LECTURING, TEACHING, GIVING LOGICAL ARGUMENTS
   Trying to influence the person with facts, counterarguments, logic,
   information or your own opinions.

6. JUDGING, CRITICIZING, DISAGREEING, BLAMING
   Making a negative judgment or evaluation of the person.

7. PRAISING, AGREEING
   Offering a positive evaluation or judgment.

8. NAME-CALLING, RIDICULING, SHAMING
   Trying to make the person feel foolish, or shaming him.

9. INTERPRETING, ANALYZYING, DIAGNOSING
   Telling the person what her motives are or analyzing why she is
   doing or saying something; communicating that you have her figured
   out, that you have her diagnosed.

10. REASSURING, SYMPATHIZING, CONSOLING, SUPPORTING
    Trying to make the person feel better, talking him out of his feelings,
    trying to make his feelings go away, denying the strength of his feelings.

11. PROBING, QUESTIONING, INTERROGATING
    Trying to find reasons, motives, causes; searching for more information
    to help you solve the problem.

12. WITHDRAWING, DISTRACTING, HUMORING, DIVERTING
    Trying to get the person away from the problem; withdrawing from the
    problem yourself; distracting, kidding him out of it, pushing the
    problem aside.

PRACTICE CYCLE #8

1. An evaluative statement is a response that:

   (a) does not help   (b) is neutral   (c) does help

2. A/an _____ is an example of a statement that does not help.

   (a) reflective listening

   (b) irrelevant statement

   (c) supportive statement

3. "Why, when I had my tooth out.....!" is an example of a/an _____.

   (a) hitch-hiking response

   (b) evaluative statement

   (c) regulatory statement

Identify which of the following are roadblocks to communication.
Mark YES if the item is a roadblock, mark NO if it is not.

_____ 4. Advising, giving solutions or suggestions.

_____ 5. Statements such as "oh" or "I see."

_____ 6. Interpreting, analyzing, diagnosing.

_____ 7. Judging, criticizing, disagreeing, blaming.

_____ 8. Repeating, in different words, what you heard the speaker say.

_____ 9. Warning, admonishing, threatening.

_____10. Ordering, directing, commanding.

_____11. Being sensitive to when the speaker wishes to terminate the conversation.

_____12. Withdrawing, distracting, humoring, diverting.

1. (a) does not help. An evaluative statement (either negative or positive) is judgmental and being judgmental is not part of responsive listening.

2. (b) irrelevant statement.   An irrelevant statement sounds as if you have not really heard what the patient said.

3. (a) hitch-hiking response   Sounds as if this person had been listening and was just waiting for the chance to jump into the conversation with her own train of thought.

4. YES

5. NO   These are door-opener phrases which facilitate further communication.

6. YES

7. YES

8. NO This is responsive learning. Good responsive listening encourages and does not block communication.

9. YES

10. YES

11. NO This too is being a responsive listener and leaving control of the conversation with the patient.

12. YES

TALKING WITH PATIENTS

"What a difference a single word can make!
With the right word, you get good results;
with the wrong one, you can create misunderstanding
and far-reaching problems."

Communication in the Dental Office

The difference between the right word
and the almost right word
is the difference between lightning
and the lightning bug.

Mark Twain

We spend over 90 percent of the nonsleeping portion of each day involved in some form of the communication process.

The effective communicator is both a sender and receiver of messages. These two roles are equally important, for it is critical that one possess skill both as a speaker and as a listener.

As a speaker you must be sure your message is understood. To do this you should:

1. <u>Send your message as clearly as possible.</u>

   a. Select your words carefully.

   b. Speak slowly, clearly and distinctly.

   c. Be sure your verbal and nonverbal messages match. Pleasant words and a sour face are confusing and offensive.

2. <u>Realize that those listening to you do not always understand your message.</u>

   a. Be alert for signs that your listener does not understand.

   b. Take steps to verify that he does understand.

   c. Be prepared to restate and clarify your message.

WORDS CAN HURT!

Intelligently managed, words are tools
as useful as a well-oiled handpiece.
Blurted out thoughtlessly,
these "wild and whirlying" things
can cut and tear and leave painful scars.[23]

Your choice of words in talking to patients is very important. The professional jargon (which you have worked so hard to master) is usually incomprehensible, even intimidating, to patients.

If you want your message to be understood, select words which the patient can understand. This requires being sensitive to the patient's level of understanding. Also remember, a high trust/low fear relationship with the patient is vital to his hearing, understanding and accepting what we say.

Even more important is our use of common words. Some words are emotionally loaded. Just hearing them alarms and upsets the patient. We can help make the patient's experience less stressful by choosing our words carefully.

Can you imagine how the patient will react if he hears the auxiliary say,

"Oh, oh!" (accompanied by a gasp that signals alarm)

"Tsk, tsk" (or any of the other sounds we use to indicate our disapproval)

"Oops!" (or any other word that slips out when something has gone wrong)

A deep sigh or yawn (indicating extreme fatigue or boredom)

WORDS CAN HURT! (continued)

Pick a Better Word

The following are examples of common words with which we do have a choice --
and that choice can make a big difference to the patient.

INSTEAD OF	TRY THIS
PAIN/HURT	DISCOMFORT
NEEDLE/SHOT	INJECTION (sleepy water for children)
PULL/YANK	REMOVE/EXTRACT
TROUBLE	DIFFICULTY
FILL	RESTORE
DRILL/GRIND/CUT DOWN	PREPARE
BASE (UNDER FILLING)	PROTECTIVE OR SEDATIVE LINING
PLATE/FALSE TEETH	DENTURE
OPERATORY	TREATMENT ROOM
WAITING ROOM	RECEPTION ROOM
DOWN PAYMENT/DEPOSIT	INITIAL PAYMENT
THE DOCTOR'S TIED UP RIGHT NOW	DOCTOR IS WITH A PATIENT
DOCTOR IS ATTENDING A CONVENTION	DOCTOR IS ATTENDING A CONTINUING EDUCATION PROGRAM

YOU-MESSAGES

*A You-message is more than the presence or absense of a pronoun.
It is a state of mind and an attitude.*

You-messages are those which explicitly, or implicitly, criticize, blame, direct or threaten. They are closely related to the "Twelve Roadblocks to Communication" which we have already discussed.

You-messages, and the accompanying tone of voice, are most commonly used in talking to children, particularly when we are scolding or directing. You-messages sometimes also creep into our conversation with adults.

They are called you-messages because the pronoun you is either actually present, as in "You should not do that!" or implied as in "Do it now!" Either way the effect on the receiver is negative and he tends to become defensive. Putting the patient, or anyone, on the defensive rarely results in effective communication.

You-messages facilitate only conflict and we need to be aware when our words and tone of voice are sending these negative signals which may interfere with our effectiveness in working with the patient.

Think back to the last time someone criticized, blamed, directed or threatened you. Perhaps you heard phrases such as "Why don't you...?" or "Would you please....?" or "If you don't...!" How did you feel in that situation? Did you feel accepted or rejected? Were you defensive or open and responsive in your communication?

How do you think the patient will feel hearing the words below? How could you phrase it better?

"YOU are late for your appointment."

"No, Mary, not that way! I'll have to show you AGAIN!"

"You will have to lose this tooth. You neglected it too long."

"Tommy, if you don't cut out sweets your teeth will all rot!"

"You MUST follow these instructions."

GIVING PATIENTS INSTRUCTIONS

Giving patient education or post-operative instructions is an important responsibility. The better you are able to do this, the more you can help the patient.

1. Keep your explanations simple. If you use unfamiliar terms, you lessen the chance that the patient will either understand or remember key points of your conversation.

2. Use short words and sentences to clarify your points and increase patient recall.

3. We remember best information which is of specific personal interest. The patient is not likely to remember a generality such as "9 out of 10 adults have periodontal disease". He is likely to remember facts specific to his case. Try to phrase your information in terms of why this is meaningful to this patient.

4. People tend to remember introductory statements and those which are emphasized best. Organize your information so that the most important point is made first and, if possible, repeated.

5. Forgetting is related to anxiety level. People often forget much of what they are told concerning instructions and advice. Simplifying terminology and actively involving the patient in a two-way discussion will improve retention and understanding.

6. Provide the patient with a written copy of instructions. These should be used as an adjunct to a personal explanation, not as a substitute. Refer to the instructions as you review them with the patient and, if appropriate, underline key points.

ANSWERING PATIENT QUESTIONS

Sometimes the patient will ask questions of the auxiliary which he would not ask the dentist. Perhaps this is because:

he is afraid of asking what may seem to be a silly question;

the auxiliary often spends more time with the patient and this is usually time when there are no hands or instruments in the patient's mouth;

the auxiliary is frequently the one to give post-operative and home care instructions;

or the patient may want more information to help him reach a decision about the doctor's recommendations for treatment and he doesn't want to take the doctor's time.

Whatever the reason, these questions provide an excellent opportunity for the auxiliary to help educate and reassure the patient.

1. In phrasing your answer, carefully select terms you are sure the patient will understand.

2. If you are not sure of the answer be honest about it. You can always offer to ask the doctor and you do not want to give out false information!

3. The patient's questions may not be directly related to his treatment or the post-operative instructions you are giving him. The patient may be asking because he is seeking reassurance that he will be alright, that he will be cared for, that help is available if he needs it.

   Be sensitive to this type of question. (Responsive listening is important here.) If the question does not seem to fit, instead of being impatient, try to understand the underlying reason.

4. We tend to reject ideas that don't fit our self-image and for this reason the patient may be having difficulty accepting the doctor's recommendation. An example is the patient who refuses to accept the diagnosis of periodontal disease because he has read somewhere that this is a disease of middle age (and he certainly doesn't consider himself to be middle-aged). Again, try to answer the questions honestly and be aware of possible underlying reasons.

PRACTICE CYCLE #9

1. List the three things necessary to sending your message as clearly
    as possible.

    _____

    _____

    _____

2. List three things you can do to be sure your message is being understood.

    _____

    _____

    _____

3. _____ are those messages which explicitly, or implicitly,
    criticize, blame, direct or threaten.

4. Technical dental terminology may be_____to the patient.

    (a) incomprehensible   (b) intimidating   (c) confusing   (d) all of these

Please complete the following by filling in the "better word".

	INSTEAD OF	TRY THIS
5.	PAIN/HURT	_____
6.	OPERATORY	_____
7.	DR. IS ATTENDING A CONVENTION	_____
8.	FILL	_____
9.	TROUBLE	_____
10.	WAITING ROOM	_____

11. You-messages facilitate only_____.

12. Receiving a you-message is likely to make me feel_____
    and this rarely results in effective communication.

13. The patient's questions MAY/MAY NOT be directly related to his treatment
    or your post-operative instructions. (Circle correct answer.)

14. List at least four points to be remembered in giving patients instructions.

    _____

    _____

    _____

15. List at least two reasons why the patient may ask a question of the
    auxiliary instead of asking the doctor.

    _____

    _____

PUT YOURSELF IN THE PATIENT'S PLACE

Pretend you are an elderly diabetic patient. You live alone and you have
just had two teeth extracted. You are worried about healing (which can
be more complicated for diabetics). You are worried about being able to
eat properly because you have to fix your own meals. You are worried about
just being able to care for yourself and wonder if help is available in
case you need it.

Now, make a list of 10 to 20 questions that this patient might ask the
auxiliary who is giving him post-operative instructions. How many of these
questions actually relate directly to the dental treatment? How many come
from your other fears and concerns?

How do you think the auxiliary can help this patient?

PRACTICE CYCLE #9   FEEDBACK

1.   SELECT YOUR WORDS CAREFULLY

     SPEAK SLOWLY, CLEARLY AND DISTINCTLY

     BE SURE YOUR VERBAL AND NONVERBAL MESSAGES MATCH

2.   BE ALERT FOR SIGNS THAT YOUR LISTENER DOES NOT UNDERSTAND

     TAKE STEPS TO VERIFY THAT HE DOES UNDERSTAND

     BE PREPARED TO RESTATE AND CLARIFY YOUR MESSAGE

3.   YOU-MESSAGES

4.   (d) ALL OF THESE

5.   DISCOMFORT   Remember we said that patients vary greatly in their experience
                  with and their response to pain. Just hearing the word can be
                  very distressing!

6.   TREATMENT ROOM   Operatory sounds like a hospital operating room and this
                      can bring forth mental images of major surgery.

7.   DR. IS ATTENDING A CONTINUING EDUCATION PROGRAM   Many people associate
                  attending a convention with going on vacation. Most dental
                  meetings have continuing education as an important part of
                  the program. Talking about these educational aspects creates
                  a far better image in the patient's mind. (It also makes him
                  aware that the doctor does indeed continue to improve and up-
                  date his skills through continuing education.)

8.   RESTORE   You <u>fill</u> a hole. The dentist is doing much more than just
               filling a hole in the tooth. He is restoring it to its
               original contour and function.

9.   DIFFICULTY   The word trouble is a lot like pain. It is emotionally
                  loaded and can be disturbing all by itself.

10. RECEPTION ROOM   We really hope the patient is not going to have to
                      wait here very long; therefore, reception room is a more
                      appropriate name.

11. CONFLICT

12. DEFENSIVE

13. MAY NOT   The patient's questions may have to do with his need for reassurance about things which are not directly related to his treatment.

14. You could have listed any four of the following:

KEEP YOUR EXPLANATIONS SIMPLE

USE SHORT WORDS AND SENTENCES

AVOID TECHNICAL JARGON

MAKE INFORMATION OF PERSONAL INTEREST

GIVE A WRITTEN COPY OF THE INSTRUCTIONS

INVOLVE THE PATIENT IN A TWO-WAY DISCUSSION

MAKE YOUR MOST IMPORTANT POINT FIRST

15. You should have listed any two of the following:

HE IS AFRAID TO ASK WHAT MAY SEEM LIKE A SILLY QUESTION

THE AUXILIARY SPENDS MORE TIME WITH THE PATIENT

THE AUXILIARY IS FREQUENTLY THE ONE TO GIVE THE PATIENT INSTRUCTIONS

THE PATIENT MAY WANT MORE INFORMATION AND NOT WANT TO TAKE THE DOCTOR'S TIME

SPECIAL PATIENTS AND SITUATIONS

DEFENSE MECHANISMS

In Section One we said that defense mechanisms are the individual's way of actively coping with a threatening, stress-producing situation. We've already talked about many ways in which we can help the patient; now let's look specifically at how we can enable him to use his defense mechanisms in a beneficial way in the dental situation.

Repression

Repression is the selective forgetting of things that are tension-producing in the individual.

It is difficult to turn this into a positive attribute in the dental situation, for this is the patient who is most likely to forget to keep his appointment or to carry through on his home care program.

Hopefully, positive dental experiences will help the patient overcome his need to repress these things. In the meantime, if the patient wants our help, we can do things such as calling to remind him of his appointment. (Many offices routinely do this for all patients.)

However, if the patient repeatedly abuses this help (by still not keeping his appointments) it may be better to tell him that we will no longer aid him in this way.

Also, it is important to have the patient retain as much responsibility as possible for keeping his own appointments. If we assume control, his excuse will be, "You didn't remind me."

After several broken appointments the doctor may refuse to reschedule the patient.

DEFENSE MECHANISMS (continued)

Deployment

Deployment is the process of getting your mind off what is going on. This is a particularly useful defense mechanism in the dental office and there are many ways in which we can help the patient with it.

1. In the reception room

    a. A warm, friendly atmosphere with pleasant background music and perhaps a bright tank of fish.

    b. Appropriate reading material such as magazines with short articles and lots of pictures. Professional journals are not appropriate.

    c. Some dentists supply cookbooks and file cards so waiting patients may copy recipes.

2. In the treatment area.

    a. A window with a pretty view and possibly a bird feeder.

    b. A mobile or small TV where the patient can see it.

    c. Keep instruments out of the patient's sight before, during and after treatment.

    d. The dentist may talk to the patient while he is giving an injection or performing other procedures. Patients may gripe, "You always ask me questions when you have your hand in my mouth!" but what they don't realize is that the dentist is doing this deliberately to divert their attention from what he is doing.

    e. When radiographs or impressions are being taken the patient may be given very specific and detailed instructions to follow. These help the patient cooperate and they take his mind off the fear that he may gag.

WHAT ABOUT PATIENT EDUCATION MATERIALS? Some dentists put them in the reception room or operatory on the theory that this is a good chance to educate the patient while his interest level is high.

Others refuse to have anything of this sort on display because they feel this is NOT the appropriate time or place (not when we are trying to divert the patient's attention). Also, they believe that these materials should be given to the patient as part of a discussion or case presentation.

DEFENSE MECHANISMS (continued)

Affiliation

Affiliation is when we are in trouble we seek the company of someone we know and trust. We have already discussed ways in which we can help the patient use this defense mechanism through both trust building and our attitudes of caring and concern.

Control

Control is the power to regulate and direct what is happening. When the patient has a high level of trust he will be more comfortable in turning over control. Also, there are ways in which we can give the patient a greater sense of controlling the situation.

1. Set up a signal system to assure the patient that treatment will stop if he indicates that he is in pain. This is usually a hand signal and often the patient will try it out at least once just to be sure the doctor will do as he promised.

2. Weiss[24] has suggested that it is helpful to get the patient actively involved in his own treatment, perhaps by asking him to hold an instrument. Weiss says, "The more a patient does for himself, the less chance he has to fret about what is being done to him."

3. Studies have demonstrated that patients who have taken responsibility in discussions involving their denture complain less than those whose dentist required no participation. A patient who leaves all decisions up to the dentist is one who may later blame the dentist for not fulfilling his expectations.

Regression

Regression is retreat to an earlier, less mature, level of adjustment. This is another defense mechanism which, hopefully, the patient will learn not to need.

In the meantime, one of the most effective ways of handling regression is to ignore it and to praise (reinforce) mature and more appropriate behavior.

THE CHILD'S FIRST VISIT

The early experiences of a young child in the dental office can be crucial in shaping his lifetime behavior and attitudes as a dental patient.

Hopefully, the child's first visit will be for an orientation session and not for treatment of a painful toothache. The primary purpose of this visit is to help the child become accustomed to sitting in the dental chair and co-operating by opening and closing his mouth on command.

This visit is planned to give the child a pleasant experience, to let him get to know the people involved, and to give him some idea of what to expect next time. The amount of treatment actually performed will depend upon the dentist's preference and the child's ability to cooperate.

Booklets, such as "Johnny's First Visit to the Dentist", are helpful in the home or school before the child actually comes to the dental office. Such materials help the child know what to expect.

Family attitudes about this first visit are also extremely important. Older brothers and sisters who are good patients can help to ease things considerably. On the other hand, parents who treat the event as "poor baby got to go to the mean old dentist" will only make things harder for all concerned.

Many dentists request that the parent remain in the reception room while the child is being examined and treated. This is because children usually behave better when mother is not around. However, the parent should be assured that the dentist will take time to talk with him at the end of the appointment.

Ideally, this policy will be explained to the parent when he calls to make the appointment. With this information, he can help prepare the child for this situation. Some offices send out a letter explaining this and other office policies prior to the first appointment.

When the child arrives at the dental office there are usually toys and books in the reception room to say "welcome". Some dentists also have a bulletin board of pictures of child patients taken after a no-cavity check-up or upon the completion of treatment. A new child seeing these pictures is reassured to know that his friends or other children have come here and had a good experience.

THE CHILD'S FIRST VISIT (continued)

When it is time for the child's appointment, the auxiliary should go into
the reception room and introduce herself to the parent and child. She
might bend or sit to be closer to the child's level. After she spends a
few moments getting to know the child (and letting him feel more comfortable
with her) she explains that she is going to take him into the treatment room
and there he will have a chance to ride up and down on a special chair,
have his teeth counted, etc.

At this point, the auxiliary takes the child's hand and they walk together
(without the parent) into the operatory. Most children will cooperate at
this point. Some will balk or hang back, but will come along with a little
firm but gentle, insistence. Others may have to be picked up and carried in;
however, this tactic is discouraged.

Some children may temporarily regress to a more infantile level of behavior.
This should be accepted, without comment, and more mature and appropriate
behavior rewarded and praised.

While the auxiliary is alone with the child she will be talking, showing him
things, and helping him relax. However, once the doctor is with the child,
the auxiliary should be quiet. Children can only pay attention to one thing
at a time -- and it is essential that the child concentrate on what the doctor
is doing and telling him.

Local Anesthesia and Children

1. Let the doctor do the talking. With good preparation and technique many
    children are not even aware that they have had a "shot".

2. During the injection be prepared for sudden movements. Calmly move your
    arm across the child's body without touching him, but in position to
    restrain movement if necessary.

3. Caution, sleeping lip. The child and his parent should be cautioned
    when the child's lip is numb. Without realizing it the child may chew
    on the lip only to discover that he has bitten himself and that it is
    very sore.

LOCAL ANESTHESIA

The use of local anesthesia can
make dentistry almost painless.
Yet many patients fear the
injection.

WHY?

The reasons are too numerous and
complex to contemplate. The important thing to realize is that we CAN
help the patient both physically and
psychologically.

Physically these things can help

1. Topical anesthesia.

2. Sharp needles of a fine gauge.

3. Anesthetic solution that is warm, not cold.

4. Slow injection technique.

Psychologically these things help

1. Do not let the patient see you preparing the syringe.

2. At all times keep the syringe out of the patient's sight
   (including when you are passing and receiving it).

3. Know what you are doing so you don't have to ask questions.
   "Dr., do you want a long needle for Mr. Smith?" may mean
   only 1 5/8" to you -- but you can be sure it will be very
   long, large and painful in the patient's imagination.

4. Learn to function effectively as part of a team so that
   the procedures go smoothly requiring minimal directions
   and discussion.

5. Recommended Reading: The Auxilary's Role in the Administration
   of Local Anesthesia.

EXTRACTIONS

We talked before about some of the psychological reasons why extractions are upsetting to patients. One of these is the very real fear of pain. Here you and the doctor can help the patient.

Local anesthesia can control the pain; however, the patient may need help in understanding what he is going to experience. According to Epstein[25] exodontia patients often have great difficulty in differentiating between the sensation of pressure and the sensation of pain.

The dentist may explain to the patient that he will be feeling pressure and motion. He may demonstrate that this does not hurt by pressing on the patient's hand.

He may also warn the patient about the sounds he will hear. The tooth is being removed from the bony jaw and bone is a wonderful conductor of sound.

How you can help

1. Know your role and be able to function smoothly.

2. Have everything in readiness and out of the patient's sight.

3. Stay with the patient prior to the procedure. Use your listening skills and follow the patient's conversational lead.

4. Be prepared for complications, such as a fractured root. Have additional instruments assembled so you can quickly bring them into use -- without fuss and scrambling through drawers. The doctor needs to concentrate on the patient, not telling you where to find instruments!

5. After the procedure you may be asked to give the patient post-operative instruction. Also, some dentists like to have a follow-up call made to the patient about 24 hours after the extraction. Often this is done by the assistant who helped during the procedure. Properly worded, this is one way of saying, "We care about you."

6. Recommended reading: The Auxiliary's Role in Oral Surgery.

THE ELDERLY PATIENT

This patient is facing many problems. Some, such as adjusting to a new denture, are directly related to his dental care. Others, including loneliness, fear of the future, concern about being able to care for oneself, reluctance to try something new, and financial worries are not directly related. However, they do affect the success or failure of the dental treatment.

There are many ways in which we can help this patient.

1. Don't rush. Allow the little extra time it may take him to walk into the operatory. Notice if he needs help into and out of the dental chair. Be ready to help; however, be aware that some people resent help they have not asked for.

2. Schedule appointments for the time of day when the patient feels best. Some patients may have to depend upon someone to bring them to the office and this, too, should be taken into consideration. If the patient tires easily, schedule short visits.

3. When making financial arrangements make certain that the patient, or person responsible, fully understands the treatment planned and expense involved. If there is third party coverage the patient may need extra help with this.

4. Many people are embarassed at being seen "without their teeth". If the patient already has a denture or partial, don't take it away before the patient meets the doctor for the first time.

5. When giving instructions be aware that the patient may have a hearing loss. Ask if he understands and have him repeat the instructions. A written copy is particularly helpful if there is someone at home who will be assisting in his care.

6. The dental appointment may be the social highlight of the patient's day. If possible, take an extra moment to ask about grandchildren, gardens or whatever is of interest to this person.

   If your doctor sees many elderly patients, it might be helpful for you to be on the lookout for announcements of programs and social services available for "senior citizens". This information could be posted in the reception room, or just brought up in conversation. Helping a lonely person find new interests and contacts could reduce the number of minor adjustments which are required primarily because the patient is lonely.

PRACTICE CYCLE #10

TRUE OR FALSE?

_____ 1. It is not necessary to take a child to the dentist until he has a toothache and requires emergency treatment.

_____ 2. Repression and regression are defense mechanisms which are not particularly helpful in the dental situation.

_____ 3. Having patient education materials in the reception room helps the patient use deployment as a defense mechanism.

_____ 4. The child's attitude toward the dentist is not affected by that of his brothers, sisters or parents.

_____ 5. The patient who is actively involved in his own treatment is less likely to fuss about what is being done to him.

_____ 6. Many denture wearers are embarassed at being seen "without their teeth" even in the dental office.

_____ 7. Regression is a retreat to an earlier, less mature, level of adjustment.

_____ 8. While the dentist is working on the child you should talk to the child and try to divert his attention from what is being done.

9. List four things which can physically help to make a local anesthetic injection almost painless.

    _____

    _____

    _____

10. _____ is the process of getting your mind off what is going on.

11. Many dentists prefer that parents DO/DO NOT accompany children into the treatment room. (circle correct answer)

12. When we are in trouble we seek the company of someone we know and trust. This is a defense mechanism known as _____.

13. _____ is the selective forgetting of things which are tension producing.

14. The higher the patient's trust level, the more likely his is to be willing to turn _____ of the situation over to those who are treating him.

15. The child's first visit to the dentist is planned to be a _____ experiment.

16. The elderly patient who is lonely may use unnecessary_____ _____ as an excuse to get attention.

17. When giving instructions to an elderly patient you should be aware that he may have a _____ loss.

18. During an extraction, the patient will feel _____ and _____; however, he will not feel _____ .

HAVE YOU FORGOTTEN HOW THINGS LOOK FROM THE CHILD'S POINT OF VIEW?

Try sitting on the floor and look around at the furniture and people. What do you see? How do you suppose dental equipment appears to a child?

While you are still on the floor have a friend stand and try to convince you to leave your mother to go with her to the treatment room. How does this "big person" appear from the child's point of view? How does your neck feel from looking up? Do you want to go with her?

How can you help a child feel more comfortable in such a situation?

PRACTICE CYCLE #10   FEEDBACK

1.   FALSE   The child should be brought to the dentist <u>before</u> he has a
              toothache and requires emergency treatment.

2.   TRUE

3.   FALSE   These materials very directly call the patient's attention
              to his impending treatment.

4.   FALSE   The child's attitude will very definitely be affected by that
              of his brothers, sisters and parents.

5.   TRUE

6.   TRUE

7.   TRUE

8.   FALSE   Do <u>not</u> distract the child while the dentist is with him.

9.   TOPIC ANESTHETIC   SHARP NEEDLES OF A FINE GAUGE

     WARM ANESTHETIC SOLUTION   SLOW INJECTION TECHNIQUE

10. DEPLOYMENT

11. DO NOT

12. AFFILIATION

13. REPRESSION

14. CONTROL

15. PLEASANT

16. DENTURE ADJUSTMENTS

17. HEARING

18. PRESSURE   MOVEMENT   PAIN

SECTION THREE: WORKING WELL TOGETHER -- THE DENTAL HEALTH TEAM

STRESS AND THE DENTAL HEALTH TEAM

The patient is in a temporary stress situation about his dental treatment;
however, the dentist and his staff work under almost constant pressure and
stress.

1.   Patients react in a wide variety of ways -- some of which are openly
     hostile. There isn't a dentist practicing who hasn't been told by a
     patient, "I hate dentists!"

2.   Dental procedures are sometimes unpleasant and occasionally painful.
     According to Walters[26], some dentists learn to accept and respond to
     this, and the patient's fear of it, in a positive manner. Others never
     form the emotional scar tissue that is required and are always **stressed**
     by the necessity of inflicting pain or by their patient's **fear of it.**

3.   Dental procedures require judgment, decision making and technical skills.
     Yet, all procedures are subject to failure due to factors beyond the
     dentist's control. As examples, an inlay may not seat properly because
     of a laboratory error, or a tooth which must be lost despite the doctor's
     best efforts.

4.   The success of a practice depends to a large degree on how efficiently
     the dentist uses his time and that of his staff. In workshop sessions
     with office teams, the primary problem most often identified is the
     tension around staying on schedule and constantly running late.

5.   The dentist has the additional responsibilities of being the leader of
     the team, working well with his staff, managing his practice and making
     business decisions which will enable him to earn a living and continue
     his practice.

6.   Each member of the team has personal stress factors in his or her life.
     Ideally, these should not be brought into the work situation; however,
     occasionally they do affect reactions during working hours.

WHAT CAN WE DO TO REDUCE THIS STRESS?

While there are many factors which increase the stress level, there are
also many things which team members can do to reduce it.

A Spirit of Cooperation

When people work together all day in a situation which is stress producing
in itself, there is bound to be some friction and conflict. However, before
anything can be done to reduce the stress level (and thereby improve working
conditions) the team members must WANT to work well together. They must be
willing to cooperate and, if necessary, to compromise.

Any staff member who is unable to work well with the others and is unable to
cooperate even after efforts have been made to resolve differences, may be
on the wrong team! She may find that she will be much happier working somewhere
else.

To be Treated with Respect

In a very unscientific study, a list of "job qualities" (with items such as
good pay, lots of coffee breaks, job security and fringe benefits) was given
to dentists, working auxiliaries and student auxiliaries. They were asked
to identify which job quality they thought was most important to the auxiliaries.
The item identified as #1, by an overwhelming majority from all groups, was to
be treated with respect.

This may surprise you, you may not even agree with it; however, it does point
out the fact that being treated with respect is important to ALL of us. Just
as we try to treat each patient with respect and dignity, team members should
strive to treat each other with this same consideration.

What Helps the Patients, Helps the Team!

When the dentist and his staff have a good relationship with their patients,
they usually also have a good relationship with each other. Patients become
more relaxed and comfortable, and they are more cooperative and easier to
work with.

The reverse of this is also true. Patients quickly sense when there is
tension, hostility or lack of cooperation among the staff. This adds to
the patient's discomfort and makes him more difficult to work with -- and
so a viscious cycle is started.

The attitudes of caring and understanding, which are so important in helping
the patient, are also important in helping the staff work effectively together.

TEAM BUILDING

The authors of Making Health Teams Work[27] identify three major factors which influence the effectiveness of a health team. These factors are: mutual goals; clear identification of roles; and problem solving skills.

Mutual Goals

This refers to having all team members working together toward the same commonly held goals. Ideally, these would have been set by the entire team. These are statements of, "Why are we here?" "What do we want to accomplish?" and "How will we go about doing this?"

We all have personal and professional goals; however, we rarely sit down and list them one-two-three. Still, being aware of them is important to us and is helpful in learning to work effectively with other team members. It is easier to be cooperative when we know we are working toward a common purpose.

Clarification of Roles

Ideally, the dentist has developed an "Office Procedures Manual" which includes clearly stated job descriptions and lists of responsibilities for each staff member.

It is your responsibility to learn, and perform, your tasks to the best of your ability. You should also be willing (and hopefully able) to aid others when they need help.

Problem Solving Skills

No matter how clearly a team understands their goals and roles, problems are still bound to arise. The manner in which these are faced and resolved is of major importance to the effectiveness of the team.

Good problem solving skills are of such importance that we are going to discuss them in detail.

Dr. Taylor has been working on three-year old Susie who screamed through the entire procedure. He was trying to save a pulpally involved tooth, but Susie's behavior made it really difficult! Mary has been working with him.

He finally decided to place a temporary sedative dressing and asked Mary to mix the material for him. She was a little slow in getting it mixed and spilled some as she passed it. Through clenched teeth Dr. Taylor told Mary, "Speed it up -- and next time be more careful!"

Mary burst into tears and rushed from the operatory ready to hand-in her resignation.

Please consider the following questions and then write what you think was going on and how it can be, or should have been, handled.

    Do you think Dr. Taylor was being unreasonable?
    Why do you think he spoke to Mary that way?
    Do you think Mary was being unreasonable?
    Did she over-react to the situation?
    Was she really the target of Dr. Taylor's anger?

You could say that both Mary and Dr. Taylor over-reacted to the situation, particularly if you think of it only as an interchange about mixing and passing material.

However, you should recognize that they are both upset after working on little Susie! Dr. Taylor has been working to save that tooth and Mary has been right in there helping him.

In such a stress situation it is no wonder that Mary was slow mixing the material, or that Dr. Taylor sounded like a bear in his response to her. Mary was not really the target of Dr. Taylor's anger, yet she took it personally and responded as if she were.

What can be done about this situation?

> Mary should realize that Dr. Taylor was upset because of Susie and didn't really intend venting all of his anger and frustration on her.

> Dr. Taylor could have found a better way of expressing his feelings.

> It would be helpful if they could find a quiet time to sit down and discuss what really happened, why it happened and how they felt. Then they should look for a way of preventing a recurrence.

> If there really is a problem about mixing that material, Dr. Taylor should plan to help Mary (or have someone else help her) until she is able to perform to his satisfaction.

PROBLEM SOLVING SKILLS

Thomas Gordon[28] has developed a simple and effective way of classifying, and solving, problems. He categorizes them in terms of: when you have a problem; when I have a problem; and when we have a problem.

When YOU have a problem

When you (the other person) have a problem and I am willing to help you solve it for yourself, I can use the reflective listening skills we discussed in communicating with patients. However, this applies only when it is your problem. Not when it is my problem. Not when it is a mutual problem affecting both of us.

In using reflective listening to help you solve your problem I listen, am accepting and reflect back your meaning and feelings. I try to avoid the roadblocks to communication. I do not control the interview, probe or give advice. I leave control strictly with you. You work to solve your own problem. You decide how much and what you want to talk about.

When I have a problem

When there is something about your behavior that is disturbing to me, but not to you, then I have a problem! In an effort to solve this problem I need to be able to communicate the information about the problem without making you defensive.

An I-message accurately and honestly reflects the effect of your behavior on me. In sending an I-message I am taking responsibility for my own feelings. This is far less threatening than suggesting that there is something wrong or bad about you because your behavior upsets me.

With an I-message, I am not telling you what to do and it does not have the negative effect of a you-message. An I-message gives you the opportunity to change your behavior without having to defend yourself. (You also have the option of not changing your behavior.)

PROBLEM SOLVING SKILLS (continued)

When I have a problem (continued)

Gordon teaches that all I-messages have three parts. In actual use this
format is cumbersome; however, it is helpful in learning to understand and
send I-messages. All three components should be present in every I-message
and they may be arranged in any sequence.

When you *(YOUR ACTION)*	I *(MY FEELINGS)*	because *(CONCRETE EFFECT ON ME)*
When you forget to send cases to the lab	*I get really nervous*	*because I am afraid the doctor will blame me.*
When you are late in the morning	*I feel really angry*	*because it throws off our schedule all day.*

You probably noticed that I-messages contain the pronoun "you".
The important difference between an I-message and a you-message
is the way it is phrased and the attitude accompanying the
statement.

When WE have a problem

The third skill involves what happens when we have a problem, one which
affects both of us. Mutual problem solving, as suggested by Gordon, assumes
that neither party is in, or wants to be in, a strict power situation in which
he or she can tell the other person what to do.

This technique has obvious limitations in the dental office where the dentist
is in an authoritarian position; however, it works well in situations such as
conflicts between auxiliaries in which both parties want to work out a solution
that is mutually acceptable to both of them, a solution in which there are no
winners or losers.

The five steps involved in mutual problem solving are: (1) stating the problem;
(2) generating possible solutions; (3) eliminating unacceptable ideas;
(4) deciding on the best solution; and (5) evaluating the effectiveness of
the solution. Rather than just discussing each of the steps, lets look at
them in the format of a fictional office situation called "Problem Solving
Staff Conference".

PROBLEM SOLVING STAFF CONFERENCE

"I am soooo angry," said Ruth through clenched teeth to no one in particular. "Sheila is late AGAIN coming back from lunch and that really messes up my schedule!" Mary, personnel director for Dr. Taylor, listened without comment. She knew Sheila, the regular receptionist went to lunch from 12 to 1 o'clock. During this time, Ruth substituted as receptionist and could not leave for lunch until Sheila returned. When Sheila finally came in, a little out of breath and laden with packages, Ruth didn't say a word. Instead, she shot an icy stare in Sheila's direction and stalked out of the room.

Irritating situations such as this often arise in a work situation. Usually they don't appear to be serious, yet they affect both morale and work. They can grow quietly until suddenly one day there is a blow-up and everyone says, "What happened?" Everything seemed to be fine." Mary was aware of the growing tension and decided to do something about the situation before it got worse. She talked to Ruth and Sheila and they agreed to put the problem on the agenda for the next staff meeting.

At the meeting, Ruth and Sheila's on-going battle over lunch hour was brought up. Mary asked if they would be willing to try a mutual, no-lose, problem solving technique she had recently learned. They agreed and Mary said she would serve as facilitator, explaining the steps as they went along.

STEP ONE: STATING THE PROBLEM

Mary asked Sheila and Ruth to each state their problem starting with "My problem is...." This is done to avoid the blaming effect of a you-statement such as, "You are always late coming back from lunch."

Sheila states her problem, "I always have to go to the bank with our daily deposit and often I have errands to do for the doctor. It is hard to get everything done in an hour and be back right at one o'clock."

Ruth states her problem, "My little boy gets out of school at one o'clock. I have to pick him up and take him to the baby sitter. The school doesn't like it when I'm late and sometimes little Jimmy cries because he worries that I am not coming." (Sheila was surprised to hear this. Ruth had never mentioned to her why she was so anxious to get out on time.)

PROBLEM SOLVING SKILLS (continued)

STEP TWO: LOOKING FOR SOLUTIONS

At this point, Mary asked everyone (even the other members of the staff) to
help in the search for possible solutions in a brainstorming session. She
put up on a big piece of paper and all suggestions would be listed without
evaluation. All kinds of ideas were encouraged, as was piggy-backing (building one idea from another). Everyone contributed and found the brainstorming
was fun. Some of the ideas seemed very practical, some were obviously not
workable, all were listed without comment.

STEP THREE: ELIMINATING UNACCEPTABLE IDEAS

Now the focus shifted back to Ruth and Sheila. Mary told them to take
turns crossing out unacceptable ideas. Sheila quickly crossed out the
suggestion that she transport little Jimmy as one more errand on her lunch
hour. Ruth crossed out the idea that she be replaced in her job. They continued
taking turns until all of the completely unacceptable ideas had been eliminated.

STEP FOUR: SELECTING AN ACCEPTABLE SOLUTION

Now everyone concentrated their attention on the remaining suggestions. They
were: (1) allow Sheila an extra half hour to take care of the bank deposit and
errands. This way she would leave at 11:30 and return promptly by one o'clock.
(2) Ruth should form a carpool with other mothers so she did not have to pick
Jimmy up at school everyday. Instead, she would only be responsible one day a
week. Adding to this, Sheila volunteered to be back early on the day Ruth
had to drive the carpool.

Ruth and Sheila agreed that these ideas combined to make up a solution they
were willing to try. The other members of the staff also felt that the change
could be carried out without disrupting the office routine.

STEP FIVE: HOW WILL WE KNOW OUR SOLUTION IS WORKING?

"How will we know this solution is working?" asked Mary. The others laughed
and said, "When we no longer have a problem!" "Fine," was Mary's reply, "and
let's set up a way of checking. If it is agreeable to you we will bring this
up again in three weeks just to be sure the solution is working."

Sheila and Ruth left the staff meeting feeling that they had found a solution which was mutually beneficial. Neither was winner nor loser. Now they were working together toward a solution which they had helped to formulate.

After three weeks they found that their solution was working so well it could be modified. Since Ruth no longer had to drive to school every day, she now had more free time and some days was able to relieve Sheila of her errands. This way they both had a more refreshing lunch hour and both benefited from the changes.

If at the end of the three weeks they had found that the solution was not working (as an example, if Ruth had not been able to form a car pool), they could have gone back and repeated the problem solving process to find a new solution.

DISCUSSION OF PROBLEM SOLVING SKILLS

The problem solving skills presented here have both advantages and disadvantages.

Disadvantages	Advantages
The techniques presented are simplistic and will not work in all situations.	These techniques are easy to learn and to use. They are proven effective. They are sufficiently flexible to be adaptable to a wide range of situations (both personal and professional).
Mutual problem solving will not work when one person is in a position of power and wishes to exercise his authority.	There are times when the dentist must use his authority and make the decisions. However, there are other times when problems, such as those involving staff relationships, which are best solved by having the people involved actively working together to find mutually acceptable solutions.

ATTITUDE is perhaps the most important aspect of applying these problem solving skills.

   All the techniques are based on the individual accepting responsibility for himself, his feelings and his actions.

   All function in an atmosphere of openness and honesty in facing problems rather than repressing them and hoping they will go away.

   All assume an attitude of cooperation and working together to find positive solutions which enable each individual to maintain his dignity and self-respect.

TRY IT OUT

The best way to test the mutual problem solving technique is to try it. If there is time in class you may want to seek solutions to the following hypothetical problem.

Dr. Cunningham gets upset when the telephone isn't answered by the third ring. He has told his staff to work out a system whereby it is answered promptly.

Carolyn is responsible for answering the phone; however, sometimes she is delayed because she is in the darkroom processing x-rays.

Marsha works chairside with the doctor. It is not easy for her to get away to answer the phone.

Rita is the circulating assistant and responsible for most of the lab work. Often when the phone rings she in in the middle of a procedure which she cannot leave.

1. List the three major parts of team building.

    _____

    _____

    _____

2. It is appropriate to use reflective listening as a problem solving tool when_____have a problem.

    (a) YOU   (b) I   (c) WE

3. Arrange the mutual problem solving steps in proper sequence.

    _____ (a) Eliminating unacceptable ideas.

    _____ (b) How will we know our solution is working?

    _____ (c) Stating the problem.

    _____ (d) Looking for solutions.

    _____ (e) Selecting an acceptable solution.

4. List the three parts of a complete "I-message".

    _____

    _____

    _____

5. List two things which were discussed that can be done to reduce stress for the dental health team.

    _____

    _____

Instructions: List the goals you think a dentist might establish for his practice.
List the goals you think an auxiliary might have for her role in that practice.
Review the two lists. Any goals which appear on both are then listed as mutual goals.

AS AN EXAMPLE: *Both dentist and auxiliary could list the goal of not routinely having to work late.*
This would then be listed as a mutual goal (one which they could work together to achieve).

THE DENTIST'S GOALS	THEIR MUTUAL GOALS	THE AUXILIARY'S GOALS

PRACTICE CYCLE #12 FEEDBACK

1. MUTUAL GOALS

    CLARIFICATION OF ROLES

    PROBLEM SOLVING SKILLS

2. (a) YOU

3. (c) STATING THE PROBLEM

    (d) LOOKING FOR SOLUTIONS

    (a) ELIMINATING UNACCEPTABLE IDEAS

    (e) SELECTING AN ACCEPTABLE SOLUTION

    (b) HOW WILL WE KNOW OUR SOLUTION IS WORKING?

4. WHEN YOU (your action)

    I (my feelings)

    BECAUSE (concrete effect on me)

5. You could have listed any of the following:

    WORK WITH A SPIRIT OF COOPERATION

    TREAT EACH OTHER WITH RESPECT

    HELP THE PATIENTS (what helps the patients, helps the team)

THIS IS THE END OF <u>PSYCHOLOGY IN THE DENTAL OFFICE.</u>

Before you proceed to the post-test on page 109, you may wish to go back
and review the instructional objectives and parts of the unit.

GLOSSARY

AFFILIATION - When we are in a stress situation we want to know that we are among friends.

ANXIETY - Vague feelings arising from threats which cannot be clearly defined.

CONTROL - The power to regulate and direct what is happening.

CULTURAL BIAS - The misunderstandings and misinterpretations caused by a member of one class not understanding a member of another class.

DEFENSE MECHANISMS - The individual's way of actively coping with a threatening, stress-producing situation.

DEPLOYMENT - The process of getting your mind off what is going on.

EMPATHY - Knowing and communicating to another that you realize how he is feeling.

EVALUATIVE STATEMENT - A response which tells the patient that you do not approve of his feelings.

FEAR - An emotional reaction to a recognized threat.

FLIGHT-OR-FIGHT RESPONSE - The body's physical response to a stress alarm.

IRRELEVANT STATEMENT - A response which is not at all related to the patient's expressed feelings.

MUTILATION - Usually the loss of a limb or extensive damage to a part of the body.

NEUROTIC - A behavioral reaction or disturbance severe enough that the person can make only a moderately successful social adjustment.

NORMAL - A level of behavior which reflects better than fair social adjustment.

PAIN - Suffering or distress of the body or mind.

PAIN PERCEPTION - The individual's psychological reaction to pain.

PAIN THRESHOLD - The point at which the individual becomes aware of pain.

PHILOSOPHY OF INDIVIDUAL WORTH - The belief that everyone, regardless of personal circumstances or qualities, has worth.

PSYCHOLOGY - The science of the mind or mental states and processes.

PSYCHOTIC - A behavior problem so severe and intense, with such deviant reactions, that social adjustment is impossible.

REFLECTIVE LISTENING - Communicating to the patient that he is being listened to and understood.

REGRESSION - The retreat to an earlier, less mature, level of adjustment.

REPRESSION - The selective forgetting of things that are tension producing in the individual.

SOCIOECONOMIC - The ethnic, cultural, family, social and economic factors which make up our background.

STRESS - Any factor which causes physical or emotional tension.

SUPPORTIVE RESPONSE - A response which tells the patient that it is acceptable to feel the way he does and offers him support.

YOU-MESSAGES - Those which explicitly, or implicitly, criticize, blame direct or threaten.

REFERENCES

1. Wm. C. Cinotti, Arthur Greider, and H. Karl Springob, Applied Psychology in Dentistry, 2nd edition, St. Louis; C.V. Mosby, Co., 1972.

2. Marvin S. Weckstein, "Basic Psychology and Dental Practice", Dental Clinics of North America, 7:4, November 1962, p. 380.

3. Alex Koper, "No Substitute for a Good Doctor-Patient Relationship" as quoted in Dental Survey, 52.7, July 1976, p. 14-18.

4. TIC, September 1975, p. 7.

5. Irving Sosnow, "The Emotional Significance of the Loss of Teeth", Dental Clinics of North America, 7:4, November 1962, p. 639.

6. Herbert M. Parker, Guide to the Psychological Evaluation of the Edentulous Patient, Jersey City; Block Drug Co., 1976, p. 3.

7. Mary E. Milliken, Understanding Human Behavior, Albany: Delmar Publishers, 1969, p. 9-10.

8. A. M. Freedman, H. I. Kaplan and B. J. Sadock, Modern Synopsis of Comprehensive Textbook Psychiatry, Baltimore: Williams and Wilkins, 1972, p. 215.

9. Sanford Plainfield and Nathan Adler, "The Meaning of Pain", Dental Clinics of North America, 7:4, November 1962, p. 660.

10. Richard S. Machenzie, "Psychodynamics of Pain", Journal of Oral Medicine, 23: 1968, p. 75-84.

11. Edwin Joy, 21st Annual Dental Seminar Day, University of North Carolina School of Dentistry, December 5, 1975.

12. Elliot N. Gale and William A. Ayer, "Treatment of Dental Phobias", JADA, 79: 1969, p. 1304-1307.

13. Forsberg and Shoeben and Borland studies as quoted in Gale and Ayer, "Treatment of Dental Phobias".

14. James R. Mullens, "Dental Fear Clinic", TIC 35:11, November 1976, p.2.

15. Loren R. Borland, "Odontophobia -- Inordinate Fear of Dental Treatment", Dental Clinics of North America, 7:4, November 1962, p. 695.

16. Kenneth R. Pelletier, "Mind as Healer, Mind as Slayer", Psychology Today, 10:9, p. 35.

17. John Powell, The Secret of Staying in Love, Niles, Ill.: Argus Communications, 1974, p. 100.

18. Edward M. Option, "Psychological Stress and Coping Process in the Practice of Dentistry", International Dental Journal, 19:3, September 1969, p. 416.

19. Borland, "Odontophobia -- Inordinate Fear of Dental Treatment", p. 692.

20. J. E. Dunlap, "Resolving Patient Fear -- I Hope You Know What You're Doing", Dental Economics, January 1977, p. 69.

21. Joyce P. Buckner, "Empathy: A Necessary Condition for Helping", The Professional Medical Assistant, IX:6, November/December 1976, p. 15-18.

22. Thomas Gordon, P.E.T. Parent Effectiveness Training, New York: Peter H. Wyden, Inc. 1974, p. 41-44.

23. Jay Weiss, "Watch Your Language! Patients Do!" Dental Management, December 1975, p. 58.

24. Jay Weiss, "Put Your Patients to Work", Dental Management, July 1975, p. 17-19.

25. Sidney Epstein, "Psychological Implications of Anesthesia", Dental Clinics of North America, 7:4, November 1962, p. 595-596.

26. Everett Walters, "How to Live with Failure and Stress", Dental Management, October 1976, p. 23.

27. Harold Wise, Richard Beckhard, Irwin Rubin, Aileen Kyte, Making Health Teams Work, Cambridge: Ballinger Publishing Company, 1974.

28. Thomas Gordon, P.E.T. Parent Effectiveness Training.

PSYCHOLOGY IN THE DENTAL OFFICE
                POST-TEST   NAME

1. _____   26. _____

2. _____   27. _____

3. _____   28. _____

4. _____   29. _____

5. _____   30. _____

6. _____   31. _____

7. _____   32. _____

8. _____   33. _____

9. _____   34. _____

10. _____   35. _____

11. _____   36. _____

12. _____   37. _____

13. _____   38. _____

14. _____   39. _____

15. _____   40. _____

16. _____   41. _____

17. _____   42. _____

18. _____   43. _____

19. _____   44. _____

20. _____   45. _____

21. _____   46. _____

22. _____   47. _____

23. _____   48. _____

24. _____   49. _____

25. _____   50. _____

PSYCHOLOGY IN THE DENTAL OFFICE POST-TEST

MATCHING

_____ 1. DEPLOYMENT   (a) The power to regulate and direct what is happening.

_____ 2. REGRESSION   (b) The selective forgetting of things that are tension producing.

_____ 3. CONTROL   (c) The process of getting your mind off what is going on.

_____ 4. AFFILIATION   (d) When we are in a stress situation we want to know that we are among friends.

                              (e) Retreat to a previous, less mature, level of adjustment.

5. The_____ is the oldest emotionally active part of the body.

    The exodontia patient may confuse_____(6) and
    _____ (7) with pain.

8. In time of stress or illness our need for acceptance and respect_____.

    (a) decreases   (b) remains the same   (c) increases

9. Pain_____is the point at which the individual becomes aware of pain.

10. Having a fish tank or bright mobile for him to watch are_____ techniques used to divert the patient's attention from what is going on.

11. Mutual problem solving is used when _____ have a problem.

    (a) you   (b) I   (c) we

12. A better word to use instead of PAIN is _____.

13. A better word to use instead of FILL is _____.

14. A better word to use instead of OPERATORY is _____.

15. Badly decayed, discolored or malpositioned teeth can severely affect the individual's _____ and psychological adjustment.

TRUE OR FALSE?

_____16. Each socioeconomic class has its own customs, standard of living and values which distinguish that class from other socioeconomic levels.

_____17. All stress is harmful.

_____18. Patients often perceive the dentist as being no more, or no less, competent than the people he selects to work with him.

_____19. What helps the patient, helps the dental health team.

_____20. In all cultures pain may be expressed openly, even dramatically.

_____21. Previous dental experience and psychological health are motivational factors which are vital in determining how the patient will behave and react in the dental situation.

_____22. Technical dental jargon may be incomprehensible and intimidating to the patient.

_____23. When the dentist is explaining something to a child, you should continue to try to divert the child's attention.

_____24. Judging, criticizing, disagreeing and blaming are roadblocks to communication.

_____25. The patient who trusts those caring for him will be more comfortable in turning control of the situation over to them.

26. Establishing a system of hand signals helps give the patient a greater sense of having_____of the situation.

The major factors in team building are_____(27), _____(28) and problem solving skills.

29. To the patient, the loss of a single tooth may be viewed as a form of

   (a) mutilation   (b) strabismus   (c) tinnitus

The eruption of the teeth increases a child's capabilities and powers because now he can_____(30), learn to_____(31) and express anger and hostility by biting and spitting.

32. The "normal" dental patient is_____during treatment, even in the presence of severe pain.

34. The behavior of the patient with_____dental fear will usually involve delaying tactics and cause the dentist lost time.

35. A_____behavior problem is so severe and intense, with such deviant reactions, that social adjustment is impossible.

36. _____behavior is a disturbance severe enough that the person can make only a moderately successful social adjustment.

The loss of teeth holds the very real threat of bodily_____(37), loss of power, and a realization of_____(38).

39. An evaluative response is_____to the patient.

   (a) not helpful   (b) neutral   (c) helpful

40. Which of the following does not describe pain?

   (a) It is an experience which demands some immediate attention.
   (b) With training we can fully understand the pain of others.
   (c) Can be defined as suffering or distress of body or mind.
   (d) Drives the individual into some behavior designed to stop it as quickly as possible.

MATCHING

_____ 41. A response which tells the patient   (a)   Reflective listening
that you do not approve of his
feelings.

_____ 42. A response which is not at all   (b)   Evaluative statement
related to the patient's ex-
pressed feelings.

_____ 43. Communicating to the patient   (c)   Irrelevant statement
that he is being listened to
and understood.

_____ 44. A response which tells the   (d)   Hitch-hiking
patient that it is acceptable
to feel the way he does and
offers support.   (e)   Supportive response

45. A "normal" dental patient _____ shows excessive fear or
anxiety during treatment.

    (a) will   (b) will not

46. A person _____ be neurotic in one area of behavior and
normal in other areas.

    (a) may   (b) may not

47. A patient's past experience with pain _____ affect his
reaction to future pain.

    (a) will   (b) will not

48. _____ _____ are the individual's way of
actively coping with a threatening, stress-producing situation.

49. To send your message as clearly as possible you should select your
_____ carefully.

50. _____ is knowing and communicating to the patient that
you realize what he is feeling.

    (a)   empathy   (b)   sympathy   (c)   psychology

PSYCHOLOGY IN THE DENTAL OFFICE
POST-TEST   NAME ____ ANSWER KEY ____

1. (c) _____   26. CONTROL _____
2. (e) _____   27. MUTUAL GOALS _____
3. (a) _____   28. CLARIFICATION OF ROLES _____
4. (d) _____   29. (a) _____
5. MOUTH _____   30. CHEW MORE FOODS _____
6. PRESSURE   may be   31. TALK (SPEAK) _____
                reversed
7. MOVEMENT _____   32. COOPERATIVE _____
8. (c) _____   33. EXTREME _____
9. (b) _____   34. MILD _____
10. DEPLOYMENT _____   35. PSYCHOTIC _____
11. (c) _____   36. NEUROTIC _____
12. DISCOMFORT _____   37. INJURY (DAMAGE) _____
13. RESTORE _____   38. AGEING _____
14. TREATMENT ROOM _____   39. (a) _____
15. SELF-IMAGE _____   40. (b) _____
16. TRUE _____   41. (b) _____
17. FALSE _____   42. (c) _____
18. TRUE _____   43. (a) _____
19. TRUE _____   44. (e) _____
20. FALSE _____   45. (b) _____
21. TRUE _____   46. (a) _____
22. TRUE _____   47. (a) _____
23. FALSE _____   48. DEFENSE MECHANISMS _____
24. TRUE _____   49. WORDS _____
25. TRUE _____   50. (a) _____